Alzheimer's & Dementia
Through the Looking Glass

Betty Weiss

authorHOUSE®

AuthorHouse™
1663 Liberty Drive
Bloomington, IN 47403
www.authorhouse.com
Phone: 1-800-839-8640

Published by AuthorHouse   07/24/2012

ISBN: 978-1-4685-9427-0 (sc)
ISBN: 978-1-4685-9428-7 (e)

Bernhardt Weiss

BELOVED

On November 26th, 1901, Dr. Alois Alzheimer described the symptoms he observed during an interview with his first patient, 51 year-old Frau Auguste Deter. Five years later he biopsied her brain, presented a report on his findings to a conference of German psychiatrists and eventually the disease came to bear his name.

"She sits on the bed with a helpless expression. What is your name? Auguste. What is your husband's name? Auguste. Your husband? Ah, my husband. She looks as if she didn't understand the question. Are you married? To Auguste. Mrs D? Yes, yes, Auguste D. How long have you been here? She seems to be trying to remember. Three weeks. What is this? I show her a pencil. A pen. A purse, key, diary and cigar are identified correctly. At lunch she eats cauliflower and pork. Asked what she is eating she answers spinach. When she was chewing meat and asked what she was doing, she answered potatoes and horseradish. When objects are shown to her, she does not remember after a short time which objects have been shown."

Betty Weiss recognizes these familiar responses from ten years of hands-on experience caring for her late husband with Alzheimer's and endless research about the disease. Writing as a layperson, she fully understands the difficulties, upheavals, sadness and frustration that come with the disease, but has neither formal expertise nor training in Alzheimer's disease nor dementia, and disclaims any and all liability arising directly or indirectly from the use of this book and anything appearing in it. Consult your own physician, attorney, accountant, financial advisor or other professionals for advice.

"Alzheimer's & Dementia: Through the Looking Glass," features over 65 easy-to-understand on-point published articles from the monthly educational, advice and news column, *All About Alzheimer's,* by Betty Weiss appearing in *Today's Senior Magazine* and will answer your questions from the first vague symptoms of the disease through all the ensuing stages. They explain the mysteries of these difficult conditions in nontechnical everyday language with never a need to refer to a dictionary, medical or scientific manual.

Continue following "All About Alzheimer's" at:

"Today's Senior Magazine"
Phone: 1-530-873-4659
Toll free: 1-877-739-1022
www.todayssr.com

ALSO BY BETTY WEISS

**"When The Doctor Says, 'Alzheimer's'—
Your Caregivers Guide to Alzheimer's & Dementia"**

Non-professionals will appreciate this easy to read informative book. Written with the layman in mind, it answers countless Alzheimer's and caregiving questions in straightforward simple language.

"Alzheimer's Surgery—An Intimate Portrait"

This is the love story of grammar school sweethearts who married, had children and built a typical American life. When the husband, a perfectly normal, intelligent, healthy, physically and mentally active man is afflicted with Alzheimer's, their world shatters.

Betty Weiss
www.caregiving4alz.com

Los Angeles, California

A Brief Basic Introduction To

ALZHEIMER'S & DEMENTIA
Through the Looking Glass

**Everyone with Alzheimer's develops dementia;
not everyone with dementia has Alzheimer's.**

Few things are more confusing than trying to clarify the difference between DEMENTIA and ALZHEIMER'S, but there is a clear distinction. A doctor might give a diagnosis of *'dementia but not Alzheimer's,'* or maybe just *'Alzheimer's'* and not mention dementia, or *'dementia of the Alzheimer's type,'* or just *'dementia,'* or *'probable Alzheimer's'*—isn't it one thing or the other? *You* want to know—*what is it!* But it's not always clear because these conditions can overlap and be so vague that even a doctor can't always know for sure.

WHAT IS DEMENTIA?

Dementia is a symptom that something is affecting the normal functions of the brain; it is not an illness or a disease in itself. Think of dementia as you would a fever. The doctor says that you have a fever—a symptom that something is wrong in your body. <u>What is causing the *fever*</u>? Is it a sore throat? Your appendix? Is it an infection, and where is the infection? Do you have the flu? It is easy to recognize a fever. The patient is warm to the touch, doesn't feel too well and a thermometer will clearly show how the patient's temperature varies from normal. We learn early on in life how to recognize a fever, but how do we recognize dementia?

Dementia is a collection of unusual behaviors that someone exhibits; an indication that physical changes have occurred in the brain. There may be trouble with language, memory loss, poor judgment, repeating things, getting lost in familiar places,

vii

inability to follow directions, unable to do simple everyday living tasks, trouble managing money; hallucinations and delusions; mood swings, agitation, hostility, combativeness; disorientation of time, people and place; neglecting safety, hygiene, and nutrition. <u>What is causing the **dementia**</u>?

These abnormal behaviors, and more, collectively known as **dementia**, create difficult problems in the home and at work. Colleagues and family get angry, they think it's being done on purpose just to annoy someone, but, no, that's not the case. Sufferers really cannot help it anymore than they can help getting a fever from an infected wound. Few think the behavior is being caused by a brain disease or other medical condition, especially since the person often looks and acts so normal.

FINDING THE CAUSE OF DEMENTIA

Hopefully, when these things occur, someone will suggest visiting a doctor. Then it is up to the doctor to find out what is causing the dementia, the odd behaviors, just as he would have to find out what causes a fever.

There would be a physical examination, blood and urine tests, he'll check coordination, balance, eye movement, speech, maybe order a brain scan. He'll give the patient a little verbal memory test and interview family members. All patient's prescriptions and dosages, over-the-counter drugs, vitamins and supplements will be looked at.

(Note: If you are going to the doctor with a loved one, remember that the patient has a memory problem and it is up to you to make certain that all such items are accurate and included.)

There are about 50 different causes of dementia, many very rare. Because some dementias are reversible, it is critical to locate the cause as soon as possible so that treatment can begin early, and since the doctor is looking for the **cause**, his examination should be very thorough so as not to miss one of the reversible ones.

By far, the most common cause of dementia is Alzheimer's disease—more or less about 60% and it is not reversible.

REVERSIBLE DEMENTIAS

Causes of dementia that can usually be identified, successfully treated and reversed:

Medications such as antidepressants, anticonvulsants, blood pressure medications, anti-anxiety medications, anti-Parkinson drugs, sleep medications and more may have interactions that cause memory problems and confusion. If more than one doctor is involved, they don't always know what others have prescribed; or a patient may be taking too much or too little of any given medication. More causes of reversible dementias:

Sluggish thyroid	Depression
Lack of sleep, sleep apnea	Alcoholism
Lack of vitamin B12	Chronic drug use
Lack of folic acid	Very high fever
Tumors that can be removed	Low blood sugar
Hormonal imbalance	Electrolyte imbalance
Lower respiratory tract infection	Urinary tract infection
Hydrocephalus, fluid on the brain	
Illness such as kidney, liver, lung disease	
Infections of the brain and spinal cord	
Head injury, either a single injury or repeated blows that a boxer may receive	

Patients can have more than one condition. In addition to an illness such as Alzheimer's, they may also have a reversible dementia and will likely do better if it is treated.

IRREVERSIBLE DEMENTIAS

It is difficult trying to sort out and distinguish the specifics of the various irreversible dementias. Even doctors get confused. To one degree or another, they all include memory problems; a decline in language and visual function; trouble with foresight, planning, anticipation, insight; learned motor skills; intelligence, judgment and behavior. They overlap from one disease to another, some symptoms never appear, the severity and presentation will vary from patient to patient, day to day, moment to moment. A medication will calm one person and send another one up the wall. Someone will progress rapidly in a year; others decline slowly over 15 or 20 years. You don't think that the most educated, brilliant, active, healthy people would be victims, but they are not immune.

Those around the person employ all sorts of plans and ideas to bring normalcy back. Just explain things, just remind them, speak louder—shout, point out their wrong thinking, draw a picture, post a sign, leave reminder clues around, buy different supplements, stop using something, start eating something, take them here and there, try physical therapy, have a friend step in, show them this and that, buy a book, do puzzles, tell them they just did it yesterday, why can't they do it now? In the end, none of this brings anyone back to who they were. Things will go better when you accept, and take the word of millions who finally realize the brain is ill, and for now, nothing can change that. Agree with your loved one, don't argue, be kind, learn to step into their world for they can no longer live in yours.

Progress is being made, but to date, there are no medications that will prevent or cure these diseases, and only a few that will help control the symptoms. Sometimes it's genetic, in the family, but most of the time, it just appears out of the blue. We can read, learn, research, keep healthy, live a good life and not stress over what we cannot control. The most well known irreversible dementia is Alzheimer's.

ALZHEIMER'S DISEASE

Alzheimer's is the most common cause of dementia in people over 65 and affects approximately 50% of those over 85. It can and also does occur in those much younger. Currently researchers do not know exactly what causes it, there is no known prevention, no cure and it is terminal.

Because symptoms and illness duration vary greatly from person to person, Lisa P. Gwyther, MSW, has famously said:

"When you've seen one person with Alzheimer's disease, you've seen ONE person with Alzheimer's disease."

In spite all that has been written about Alzheimer's, it still remains one of the all-time mystery maladies. If you want to study and learn about the technical information known about it throughout the medical community, there are thousands of websites and libraries full of books to research. This book, however, is designed to give those suddenly thrust into the world of Alzheimer's a simple, general, accurate, fast-track, non-scientific, non-medical, non-technical overall layman's view of the disease. Hopefully it will erase the misinformation that too many believe and help them to better understand the reality of what they are dealing with.

"ALL ABOUT ALZHEIMER'S"

REPRINTED FROM
TODAY'S SENIOR MAGAZINE
SEPTEMBER 2006 TO MAY 2012

TABLE OF CONTENTS

AN INTRODUCTION

Until my husband came down with Alzheimer's, I knew little about it and had scant interest in learning. So someone forgets—big deal. I forget things all the time, my car in a parking garage; words that elude me, only to pop into my head hours later. I lose my keys, glasses, checkbook, important papers, any item smaller than a Clydesdale. Most of the time I can't remember birthdays, names, appointments—once I forgot to go in for surgery! Standing in the middle of the bedroom, I wonder why did I come in here? I go to the store for bread and come home with everything but.

Let me assure you, I do not have Alzheimer's and neither do you if you're the same way—and, no, it doesn't start out that way. These normal daily memory lapses are because some of us are easily distracted—especially in our modern society. We keep calendars, make lists, carry day planners, BlackBerries and cell phones that have all sorts of little alarms and reminder gadgets—you can even get a service to phone and remind you of things. Who remembers more than a few phone numbers anymore? Speed dial does it for us. We rely less and less on our own mental memories, and that's not good. Yes, sometimes the elderly get a little forgetful, but that's not always Alzheimer's either.

Alzheimer's is often called the 'Disease of Forgetting,' but that's misleading and frightening because normal people forget things all the time and then remember them later. With Alzheimer's, the victim doesn't remember later because the memory is lost, it doesn't exist anymore. And if it doesn't exist, it cannot be retrieved. The one Alzheimer's blessing, if you can call it that, is that patients don't remember that they can't remember. It is left for those of us who love and care for

1

them to watch that tragedy. And, yet, there are times when the patient remembers, appears to be perfectly normal. You think that maybe it isn't Alzheimer's after all.

Alzheimer's is extremely difficult to diagnose. Doctors do a variety of verbal, physical, blood and urine testing and brain scans, mostly to rule out anything else that may be causing unusual behaviors. They are looking for brain tumors, stroke, other brain diseases, excessive drug or alcohol use, lack of certain vitamins or supplements, side effects of medications, infections, head injury, any bodily illness such as kidney, liver or lung disease. If they can't find anything else, they often give the diagnosis of 'probable' Alzheimer's. How can it be 'probable,' isn't it either one way or the other? Well, not exactly, these methods are considered 80% to 90% accurate. The only 100% certain diagnosis is through a brain biopsy, usually done at autopsy—hence the 'probable' modifier.

A new brain scan is said to be able to track the progress of Alzheimer's from the very beginning. That's good, because the sooner it is detected, the sooner medications and monitoring can begin and, hopefully, delay the progression. Otherwise, there is no way that anyone—doctor or layman—can possibly see the very beginning symptoms of Alzheimer's. They are too gossamer, too vague, too easily dismissed as aging, stress, depression.

The disease attacks the brain decades before the difficult behaviors come roaring out. Sometimes colleagues at work are the first to notice. A worker who never missed a thing becomes a bit forgetful and confused. Since it's not all the time, others will often cover the mistake. Few think it's a brain disease—maybe it was just a fight with the wife or financial concerns.

Or question Mom's family members and many will admit that from time to time, she has seemed a bit forgetful. But it can't be Alzheimer's, she's just getting old, isn't that normal? Most of the time, yes. Short-term and remote childhood memories aren't usually affected by aging. Forgetting a word is just a 'hiccup' in the aging memory, it will often be recalled later. Frustrating, but not usually serious.

Memory loss that is not a part of aging may be trouble learning new things, forgetting how to do things done many times before, repeating phrases or stories in the same conversation, problems handling money, not being able to keep track of daily happenings. A doctor's visit may be in order.

CAUSES

Exactly one hundred years ago, in 1906, a woman died in Frankfurt-am-Main, Germany. Her name was Frau Auguste Deter and she had been admitted to the Municipal Mental Asylum there in 1901, when she was 51. The senior physician at the hospital was Dr. Alois Alzheimer. By the time she died five years later, Dr. Alzheimer had taken a position at the Anatomical Laboratory of the Royal Psychiatric Clinic at Munich University. Her brain was sent to him for examination.

His findings of "plaques and fibrules" (now called plaques and tangles) formed his hypotheses that there was an organic cause for the condition. Plaques are clumps of protein fragments that accumulate outside of the brain's nerve cells. Tangles are twisted strands of another protein that form inside brain cells. This was not a new discovery, but a paper he presented, November 4, 1906, about Frau Deter at the 37th Conference of Southwest German Psychiatrists was the first to describe a clinical case of dementia. Eventually, his name became attached to the disease.

He described Frau Deter's symptoms, including disorientation, aphasia (problems with language), auditory hallucinations, paranoia, unpredictable behavior, and pronounced psychosocial impairment; the same things families deal with today. Any social or environmental context to explain her condition was never addressed.

In spite of what we've learned in the past century, Alzheimer's root cause is still a mystery. Many theories abound, but the same plaques and tangles continue to appear. I believe Alzheimer's has been around for hundreds of years, certainly longer, so I don't think it's anything in our modern life style that

4

brings it on. Frau Deter did not drink soda from an aluminum can, she did not consume fluoride, saccharine, processed foods, eat veggies with pesticides or have mercury fillings. She was one of countless patients in asylums at the time, and it is hardly a stretch to believe that most suffered a variety of brain diseases, other illnesses or injuries.

Alzheimer's is called a 'disease of aging,' but that's not wholly accurate. Alzheimer's attacks the brain decades before overt symptoms occur, it's already lingered for a long time—silent, unseen, undetected, ignored. Cells were dying while the patient was young with little effect on daily living. It appears to start with aging because, today, we live long enough for it to become full blown—too many cells are finally lost. Generations ago people who had it died young, well before it could show up.

Nor do I subscribe to the 'use it or lose it' theory. Ask anyone whose Mom has Alzheimer's and you'll likely be told that Mom was an unusually bright woman with an important job, busy at church, active in organizations, well groomed, healthy, funny, a college graduate. Few ever say Mom was a dullard, a dropout, a couch potato who spent her days watching TV munching chocolates.

My husband was a healthy, brilliant engineer who ran his own business designing and manufacturing units for all the early space shots. Incredibly active, mentally and physically, he 'used it' all the time. Hoping to avoid Alzheimer's, people do crossword puzzles, take classes, learn tricky dance steps, gulp supplements, exercise regularly—all to the good—but does that really work? So, if it's not what we eat, do or don't do, a college education, microwaves, high-tension wires—what does cause this mysterious malady? If only we knew.

Late-Onset or Sporadic Alzheimer's is the most common type of the disease and affects about 90% of those with Alzheimer's over the age of 65. Also, about 50% of all people over the age of 85 suffer from it and the cause is unknown. Of the hundreds of people in my husband's extended family, only one elderly woman was known to have dementia. Was it Alzheimer's? Possibly—no one knows.

Early-Onset Alzheimer's strikes people younger than 65 and affects only about 5% to 10% of those with the disease. It can develop between the ages of 30 and 40, but that's uncommon. Usually it occurs in people in their 50's. A doctor I know has told me that his youngest early-onset Alzheimer's patient is 29. As a layman, I now believe that's what my husband probably had, he was very young, but I just thought his odd behaviors, from time to time, were because of stress—whatever, I never recognized any of it as a brain disease.

Familial Alzheimer's is also part of early-onset Alzheimer's, but it differs in that about half of early-onset patients have inherited certain genes that run in the family and may mutate and lead to Alzheimer's. You can get tested, but even if you have these family genes, you may never get Alzheimer's. Problems with testing are that you could be denied insurance, job opportunities, (medical records can be subpoenaed), and maybe impact serious relationships.

My husband does not seem to have fit into any of these categories. It's a little of this and a little of that, it certainly has not been known to run in his family. It's all very fluid, much still needs to be learned, but for sure, he had Alzheimer's.

My layman's opinion is that many people carry recessive genes connected to Alzheimer's that may lie dormant throughout life—or until something awakens them. Surprisingly, many of us have plaques and tangles in our brains, but we never get Alzheimer's. Go figure.

DEMENTIA OR ALZHEIMER'S?

**Everyone with Alzheimer's develops dementia;
not everyone with dementia has Alzheimer's.**

You finally got past the denial and took your loved one for a diagnosis. Was it *'dementia,'* *'possible Alzheimer's,'* *'dementia of the Alzheimer's type,'* or just *'Alzheimer's'?* The possibilities are endless.

Dementia is the key word here. Dementia is neither a disease nor an illness. It is a term describing symptoms that may include repeating things, language problems, getting lost in familiar places, inability to follow directions, disorientation about time, people and place; neglecting personal safety, hygiene, and nutrition; unable to solve simple tasks, trouble making change, mood swings, agitation, etc. It was these odd behaviors, the dementia, that ultimately sent you to the doctor. You may have thought it was Alzheimer's, and you could be right. Alzheimer's is the major cause of dementia, but it might be something else. Dementia can be caused by Parkinson's, Huntington's, kidney, liver, heart or lung disease; strokes, tumors, reactions to meds, infections, diminished oxygen, excessive alcohol or drug use, head injury, nutritional deficiencies, fluid in the brain, etc.

Because some dementias are reversible, it is critical to find the cause. Dementia is not part of normal aging. You can think of dementia as a fever. Is it being caused by the flu, an infected toe, an appendix attack or something unknown? You have to find out. Dementia, in and of itself, like a fever, is a symptom.

Alzheimer's, however, is definitely a **disease.** Besides tangles and plaques, the Alzheimer's markers found in the brain at autopsy, there are other brain changes. Nerve cells vital to mental abilities die. Connections between cells fail. Lower levels of some brain chemistry may impair language, thought, and memory. Our brains also control numerous body functions we are unaware of—circulation, breathing, blinking, swallowing saliva, digestion, heartbeats, etc. Eventually, those things are also affected. Alzheimer's is a terminal disease. When my husband's brain could no longer control his automatic breathing, he was given oxygen to insure a peaceful passing. But his brain had simply stopped his breathing and there was nothing to be done. Scientists do not know what causes Alzheimer's. A few meds may delay its progress in some people, sometimes, but there is no cure and no way to halt its ordained destruction. It is not a part of normal aging.

A diagnosis of Alzheimer's is sad and frightening. But usually it is very slow moving and many years of normal, happy living often lie ahead. On average, patients live about seven years after diagnosis, but it is not uncommon to live another twenty. My husband lived for ten, but I know he had it many years before going to the doctor.

Something important to understand and remember. Because people with dementia and Alzheimer's may have many lucid moments, because they look the same and often act normally, those around them tend to think there is nothing wrong, they can understand and remember when they want to. They're putting on an act, looking for attention. If Dad was able to lock the gate yesterday, he can certainly do it today! But think of memory as a sand castle at the ocean's edge, perfectly fine until the tide changes. A little lap of water nibbles away at the outside edge, no one notices. Later, water comes up at another place, takes a bit more but leaves most of the castle still intact. Parts gone with the receding tide are lost forever—and you don't know exactly which ones they are. As the castle slowly disappears, so does the ability to understand. So, yelling at those with dementia, insisting they remember, explaining this and explaining that, only bewilders them and frustrates you. As cells die, their reality changes; it is no longer the same as yours. It takes some doing, but learn to deal with whatever outrageous things they say; they truly believe what they believe. You cannot restore functions that no longer exist, but you can keep your home as calm as possible, move into their reality, understand what it's like for them, give lots of love, and make things easier. No small challenge.

If you feel uncomfortable with your doctor, don't hesitate to find another. Most doctors are never taught much about dementia. A neurologist specializing in the brain or a geriatrician is a good place to start. You have a long road ahead and you'll need all the experience, expertise and support that a knowledgeable physician can provide. If there is a large university or training hospital nearby, find out if they have some type of Alzheimer's or Memory Clinic.

WARNING SIGNS

For the most part, there is no clear-cut line between normal aging changes and warning signs of Alzheimer's. Too often the early signs of Alzheimer's are not easily recognized or taken seriously, even by doctors. It's expected that some people get a little pixilated as they age—it's no big deal. But sometimes it *is* a big deal—a very big deal, and the family that takes a loved one, *old or not so old*, to their physician at the first vague signs is well advised. Common symptoms for Alzheimer's could also be symptoms for so many other things. Sometimes a diagnosis of Alzheimer's is made, and then changed a year or two later to something else—it can be that elusive. It is important to be aware of these typical warning signs and not think that they are just normal aging.

1. **Memory loss:** On occasion, almost everyone will forget an appointment, names and phone numbers but will eventually remember later; the Alzheimer's patient will forget more and more often and not remember things later because the memories get erased. If erased, they cannot be retrieved. They will not even remember that they forgot.

2. **Difficulty performing familiar tasks:** Things always done automatically become impossible. Making a sandwich is too confusing; how many slices of bread, do you use a knife or a spoon, does the lettuce go on top, how do you get the meat inside? People with Alzheimer's will be unable to operate household appliances safely, make a phone call or play a favorite game.

3. **Problems with language:** From time to time, we all forget words but they eventually come back; Alzheimer's

patients not only forget words for simple objects, they often substitute another word that is close but incorrect. A 'car' can become a 'bus'—a 'fork' will be called a 'dish'—a 'toothbrush' will be 'that thing for my mouth'.

4. **Disorientation to time and place:** It's normal to forget the day of the week, even forget where you're driving, but those with Alzheimer's can get lost on their own street, even in their own house when they can't find the bathroom. They don't know how they got someplace and have no idea how to get back home.

5. **Poor or decreased judgment:** No one always has perfect judgment but Alzheimer's patients dress without regard to the weather, wear two or three shirts, set out for work with pants over their pajamas, wear underwear on top of street clothes. They easily lose money or give away large amounts to someone on television, a telemarketer, or paying bills they don't owe.

6. **Problems with abstract thinking:** Numbers become very confusing; they cannot remember the value of what a number represents. Alzheimer's patients won't be able to make change, figure out a receipt, how to leave a tip or balance a checkbook.

7. **Misplacing things:** We all lose things but usually find most of them. However, it is especially difficult with Alzheimer's patients who often 'hide' things—that you may never find—and then accuse others of stealing their things. They put a shoe in the microwave, the scissors in the refrigerator.

8. **Changes in mood or behavior:** Everyone has occasion to feel sad or moody, but those with Alzheimer's can swing rapidly from happiness to tears or calm to anger—and often for no apparent reason.

9. **Changes in personality:** Sometimes, as people age, they may get a little sweeter or nastier, but Alzheimer's people often get confused, suspicious and fearful. The most independent can turn very dependent and attach themselves to one particular person, usually the one closest in their life—a spouse or an adult child.

10. **Loss of initiative:** On occasion everyone gets bored and tired of the same routine—housekeeping, work, social events—same people, same things, same activity, same conversations, but with Alzheimer's the patient may become very passive, seemingly unable or unwilling to do any normal activities, just sitting in front of the television—not really watching or involved in what's showing—or sleeping the time away.

Many healthy people are unable to remember certain things as they age, but Alzheimer's symptoms are much more severe than simple memory lapses. Alzheimer's is progressive, the symptoms worsen over time. How fast the disease progresses and the pattern of symptoms that occur, varies by the individual.

TRAGEDY AT THE SANTA MONICA
FARMERS MARKET

When an 86-year-old man ran down people with his automobile at the Santa Monica Farmers Market in Southern California, many believed he had to have been demented. On TV, I recognized his same vacant smile I had seen countless times on my husband and others with dementia when they had no idea what was happening around them. They are very good at keeping up appearances, hiding problems. Imagine being in a roomful of people playing a game and you have no idea who they are or what the game is, so a friendly smile, a friendly greeting, saying whatever seems appropriate will take you a long way. Few notice you're not really involved in what is happening; most of the casual things we say to each other are so much chaff anyway.

I didn't hear anything about the driver possibly having any cognitive impairment, maybe an illness like Alzheimer's, medication reactions, a mini-stroke, and my writing about it is not meant in any way to defend or excuse him. I wasn't at the scene or the trial. Emotions ran high, witnesses saw what they saw. In October, he was found guilty of vehicular manslaughter negligence. In November he was sentenced to five-years probation, the judge noting he *should* serve jail time, but his failing health precluded that. I just want to suggest the possibility that well-meaning people may all see the same event in a different light.

One witness talked about seeing the man smirk. But I didn't see that smile as a smirk. To me, it was a way to cover up confusion. Attorneys for the driver fought to keep him out of the courtroom, one wonders why. Witnesses said he did it deliberately, avoided parked cars, hitting people instead, told of his coldness, lack of concern and even his arrogance after the crash. In court, he had no response to a picture of his car with bodies still on it—but if demented, he couldn't connect such a photo to himself and what happened. Lack of remorse, getting angry, displaying a flat response, being unable to apologize are all typical of dementia. Jurors thought he had time to stop, but he couldn't if he had any mental impairment. They rejected the idea that people can freeze on the gas pedal instead of the brake, but it happens. We've all seen photos of a car crashing off a parking structure, into a swimming pool, a storefront, mowing down people at a bus stop. Why didn't they just stop!

People see a scrubby man mumbling and pacing on a street corner and think, correctly, that for one reason or another he is demented. They imagine uncontrollable, demented people confined to a care facility. But most people with dementia are not in such places; they live in the homes of ordinary people, in your town, being cared for by family that often covers for them. You have no idea there's any problem when you see them. They can be well groomed, personable, smiling, often well spoken. No one realized anything was wrong with my husband. When I finally had to place him in a facility, everyone said, "I didn't see anything wrong." I am reminded of President Reagan's strolling in a park, so neat and clean, smiling—yes, the smile—stopping when someone asked for a photo together. But few recognized the dementia that Alzheimer's ravaged upon him. That was seen and tended to only by his family and caregivers.

Countless families have no idea anything is wrong with a loved one and far too many are still driving! They have diminished capacity behind the wheel and it is so subtle, so vague that few see it. Families choose denial or truly believe quirky behavior is just normal aging. Even if they do see it, they often ignore it for years.

It's too hard to confront a parent or spouse; it's fear of finally acknowledging that something is terribly wrong; fear of the unknown—and the known. It's being embarrassed—no one wants to admit something is wrong with the mind. It's too heartbreaking to take away someone's independence, and since Mom never drove, who's going to take her to the market?

STAGES

Few people know what to expect when there is a diagnosis of Alzheimer's. Many have heard it's about forgetting, that you can forget your own children or where you live. But most believe there's no way you can really forget your children—not me, not us, not mine. It is almost impossible to understand that someone can forget how to chew, put on a jacket, open a window, but these things happen.

In an effort to understand what to expect, experts have devised stages of symptoms as they usually occur. These stages are not in locked boxes, they often spill over into each other and some things never happen. But they are a useful frame of reference for families and doctors. Some individuals stay in certain stages for a longer or shorter period of time and they can move slowly from stage to stage or rapidly; there are no exact timetables. The duration of these stages, collectively, can easily vary anywhere from three to twenty years.

The **Seven Stages of Alzheimer's** were developed by Barry Reisberg, M.D. and are based, in a general way, on the pattern of progression that corresponds to brain cell degeneration that typically begins with damage to cells involved in learning and memory, gradually spreading to every aspect of thinking, judgment and behavior, and eventually to the cells that control and coordinate all unconscious movement like breathing, heart beat, digestion, blinking, swallowing saliva, etc.

Stage 1: **No impairment**.

Stage 2: **Very mild cognitive decline** is easily confused with normal aging. Problems are not evident to family, friends and even doctors; but patients will feel they are having memory lapses and forgetting familiar words and locations of ordinary items.

Stage 3: **Mild cognitive decline** is noticed by co-workers, friends and family. Patients have trouble remembering names of newly introduced people, losing valuable objects, and a decline in their ability to plan and organize.

Stage 4: **Moderate cognitive decline** brings the inability to remember recent events; cannot do simple arithmetic like counting backwards from 100 by 7's; unable to plan meals, pay bills, make change or do marketing; and losing memory of personal history. They may seem subdued and apart from others during social gatherings or mentally challenging situations.

Stage 5: **Moderately severe cognitive decline** will have major memory gaps and deficits in cognitive function. Patients are unable to recall important personal details such as phone number and address, but will still know some things about themselves and names of spouse and children. They will be confused about the day, date or season, need help with selecting appropriate clothing and some other day-to-day activities. They are still able to eat and use the toilet by themselves.

Stage 6: **Severe cognitive decline** will show significant personality changes and more memory difficulties. Individuals need extensive assistance with common daily activities. They lose awareness of recent experiences; do not remember personal history correctly, forget name of spouse—but usually still remember their own name, can generally distinguish between familiar and unfamiliar faces; without supervision will put clothes on incorrectly and backwards, shoes on wrong feet; sleep patterns become interrupted; need help with all phases of toileting and increasing urinary and fecal incontinence; become suspicious, delusional, have hallucinations, can be compulsive with repetitive physical behaviors, and tend to wander and get lost.

State 7: **Very severe cognitive decline** is the final stage. Individuals lose the ability to speak, although words or phrases may occasionally be heard, need help with eating, unable to walk without assistance, to sit without support or hold head erect, unable to smile, reflexes become abnormal, muscles grow rigid and chewing and swallowing is impaired.

Sometimes doctors use **Three Stages** but they follow the same general progression of loss. Generally the **Early Stage** (1) affects job performance, making bad decisions, loss of initiative; **Middle Stage** (2) brings refusal to bath, repetitive statements, problems with reading; **Late Stage** (3) has weight loss, unable to recognize self in mirror and can't communicate verbally.

Keep in mind that stages overlap, some things never happen and not all individuals do all the same things at the same time. Remember that all normal people have memory lapses and other such problems from time to time, don't jump to the conclusion that it is always Alzheimer's.

HALLUCINATIONS & DELUSIONS

So many things about Alzheimer's are disturbing to our senses—surprising, frightening, unexpected, bewildering. You walk into the bathroom to find your husband is laughing and talking to his reflection in the mirror. He turns to tell you 'that's sure a nice fellow I've been talking to' and your heart sinks. He can no longer recognize himself in a mirror, or you if you are standing next to him, so he talks to the nice man.

It scares you when he yells at someone you can't see, or has a conversation with a figurine. Your first reaction, naturally enough, is to tell your loved one that there is no one to yell at, the figurine is not real—and in return, he is likely to tell you that it *is* real, because to him it is—as real as the things you yourself see.

Hallucinations are things an individual will see, hear, smell, taste or feel through his senses and they are absolutely real to him. But it's all a false perception caused by changes in the brain. It does no good to tell him otherwise. He may agree for the moment, but it will happen again and again. The changes in the brain cannot be reversed and restored. If the hallucinations are not frightening to the patient, and if you can get your mind around the idea that they are not frightening to you either, then it is good to just agree, to go along with whatever your loved one is seeing or hearing. Go into his reality for the moment. Tell him that *was* a nice man (in the mirror), that you are happy he had such a good visit. You can even ask him to tell you all about it. Better to validate the experience; arguing about it will only cause frustrations for both of you.

If your loved one has an hallucination that frightens him, then you have to take a different tack. I have talked directly to

19

something only my husband saw, told it to 'go away' to 'get out of the house.' It usually worked. You have to reassure your loved one that he is safe and everything is alright. You won't let anything bad happen. Yes, you are telling a lie to ease the situation, just as you tell a small, frightened child that Mommy will always be here. You can't guarantee it, but you go with the odds. Again, you can ask him to talk about it, commiserate with things like 'gee, that really sounds bad, but it's gone now, let's have some ice cream.'

Everyone on occasion 'sees' a face in a cloud, a curtain, a shadow, but Alzheimer's patients cannot understand that it is only an illusion. You can try to modify the environment by keeping areas well lit to avoid shadows, cover mirrors, rearrange curtains, and draw shades at night to avoid reflections in the windows. Again, you can try to divert your loved one's attention with an extra hug, a short walk, music, sorting coins or buttons, hold hands, enjoy the moment and have some hot chocolate.

Delusions are something else and often harder to deal with. These are not things they 'see' or 'hear,' but ideas that get into their heads and it can be impossible to get them out. They often become suspicious, accuse others of stealing, someone is spying, their food is poisoned. Your loved one may accuse you of not being you, call you an imposter and say that this is not his house. The more you try to reason with him that you are really you and this is his house, the more he will accuse you of lying.

If he insists that something has been 'stolen,' help him look for it; say it's been lent to a friend, it's at the cleaners, whatever works for the moment. My husband accused me of being unfaithful and when I said, 'but I'm right here with you' he shot back 'oh, no, you're not!' This was hard to combat because I could not agree and could not deny without escalating things and being called a liar. So I'd try, somehow, to accept responsibility without admitting guilt, and if you think that it's all impossible, you're right—*it is impossible*—it's Alzheimer's.

PLACEMENT OR HOME CARE

People often ask how will they know when it's time to place an Alzheimer's loved one. There is no 'set' time. Placement will not improve the patient's condition. The disease will progress at its determined pace whether in the home or in a facility, if cared for by a family member or a staff of professionals. Many caregivers are like new mothers, believing that 'no one can take care of my baby/my Mom as well as I can.' They think placement will make Mom worse, it'll kill her. Unless it is a snake pit of a facility and no one is making regular visits, that's not likely to happen.

Few understand how daunting it is to take care of someone all alone with Alzheimer's. The main reason for placing an Alzheimer's patient is when you cannot get enough in-home help and there is no one in the family healthy enough, young enough, well enough, strong enough, willing enough to continue unrelenting 24/7 caregiving, doing the work of a professional staff all alone for years with no end in sight. Fifteen percent will die before their contemporaries; far too many die before the patient they are caring for; forty-three percent will fall into a clinical depression that can linger for years, even after the loved one dies; and elderly caregivers with their own chronic illness have a sixty-three percent higher mortality rate than their non-caregiving peers. Placement is really to save caregivers because their well-being is every bit as important as that of the patient but is too often put on the back burner. Further, it can crack a marriage wide open and take parents away from their primary task of being there for their children. So it's a dilemma few want to face.

Placement is most often harder on the caregiver than the loved one. Normally, a patient will adjust within a month or so, but the caregiver can't get over the guilt, visits all day every

21

day and talks about bringing Mom or hubby back home. They worry about the promise made to never place Mom in a home, the marriage vows they really want to keep. It's a good guess that most Alzheimer's patients in a care facility had a loving caregiver who never-ever meant to stop being the one and only true home caregiver. But the hard facts of life are that life, itself, intrudes on all our plans. We take a vow when we're twenty to cherish in sickness and in health, but fifty years later that young, healthy, strong, confidant bride is a great-grandmother with her own aging problems. Or you promised your Mom that you'd never put her in a nursing home, but now you have one child in college, a couple still in high school; increasing rifts in your marriage and your own health is neglected because you just don't have time for everything and everyone.

Some indications that a caregiver needs significant additional assistance and might consider placement: Not sleeping; crying uncontrollably; not getting things done; anger at and hitting your loved one; relationships with others deteriorating; increased drinking, smoking, use of drugs; poor appetite or uncontrolled eating; retreating into yourself; thinking no one else can adequately care for your loved one and refusing help; always feeling sorrow, guilt or hopelessness; patient's health is declining and needs constant medical care; your own health is deteriorating; feeling like you're living in limbo; you keep thinking of getting just a little break; the idea of a care facility is not as unacceptable as it was in the beginning; **family, friends, doctors and other medical personnel are recommending placement to you.**

Certainly, caregivers need to make their own choice between placement and continued home care. But a vow to take care of someone does not mean you have to do it all alone at home 24/7 for years until you drop. It still fulfills your pledge if you get help in the home, turn to family and friends, and maybe it means placement. Placement is **not** abandonment, it doesn't mean failure; it's **accepting** reality. Your loved one will still require your **active** care participation—it's not a free ride.

22

BATHING

As Alzheimer's progresses, the most fastidious fashion plate can become a slob *extraordinaire*. Removing dirty clothes is a wrestling match; bathing, a battle royal. Your loved one is perfectly happy and content 'as is,' threatens you if you get too close and refuses to bathe.

Alzheimer's patients can be very sensitive to loud noise, especially several noises at once. Bathing becomes frightening because of echoes off tiles in the stall shower, background noise of a radio or TV, screeching children and clanging kitchen sounds are too much. When helping with bathing, speak normally, try not to yell. Bathrooms have a lot going on: running water, flushing toilets, temperature changes, heaters, drafty windows, steam, fans, vents and sometimes, strange people. Water is coming down on their head, something is being rubbed into their hair, it's all slippery, they're afraid of falling. Glasses and hearing aids have been removed; they can't hear and see clearly, something is dripping into their eyes. Mirrors add the belief that people are watching, there's no privacy—they won't let you wash them 'down there.'

There are problems with Alzheimer's vision. A bathroom with white tile floor, tub and shower confuses the patient. A change in depth perception makes them unable to distinguish where the white tile floor ends and the door to the white tile shower begins. If floor, tub and shower tiles are the same color, put a different colored rug or towel at the tub or shower entrance so they can distinguish one thing from the other. Water in a tub can look like there's no bottom—it's terrifying. If possible, fill the tub after they get in, four to six inches is enough. And then, for whatever reason, they are frequently afraid of water.

Before beginning a shower or bath, get the house quiet, although soothing background music may help. Have everything set up beforehand so there's no standing around half dressed, waiting. The bathroom should be the right temperature, tumbling a robe and towel in the clothes dryer for a few minutes is comforting. A shower chair, if wanted, is available at medical stores. Use a handheld showerhead so you can control the off-on water flow and move around the body. Test water temperature first. Try turning off the shower before your loved one gets in, it may be less disturbing if one does not have to step in under the water. Have all fresh clothes laid out and dirty ones out of sight. Putting a book, toy or anything in their hands to distract them will help you get clothes off easier.

Stick-on decorations and mats on the shower and tub floors are helpful. Install handrails early on so there is time to learn to use them. You can let your loved one wear underwear or a wrap-around towel for modesty while bathing. Leave glasses and hearing aids on if possible. Pleasant smelling gels with a net sponge are nice. Try gentle baby shampoo. If you can't wash their hair, use a dry shampoo. There are dry and no-rinse shampoos and body baths that can be left on, all available at your local stores or look on a computer.

You can step into the shower first and coax a loved one in, stay there if necessary. Give them something to keep their hands busy, a rubber ducky, a plastic anything, a washcloth so they can 'help' wash themselves—but not a bar of slippery soap. Tell them where you are going to wash next. Although you will want to work quickly, don't rush your loved one. Responses and understanding are getting slower.

For tub baths, again, sprayer and shower chair if wanted, plastic floor mat and, repeating, not too much water, four to six inches is enough; sometimes it helps to let them see the water going into the tub rather than having it already there, or let them get in before filling the tub. Remember handrails to help getting in and out. No one needs to bathe every day, once a week is more than enough with a sponge bath between, maybe in bed—but don't let them see the basin of water—sometimes water frightens them. A treat is always good. Promise, 'As soon as we finish, we'll drive over and get chocolate ice cream.'

Sometimes only a sponge bath is possible, but do try to keep face, hands, feet and genitals clean. It is often difficult for one person to do these things alone. Call an agency, ask around at Alzheimer's organizations, support groups, care facilities and senior centers for people who come to the house just to do the bathing, it still may take two of you. Never leave your loved one alone in the tub or shower! Whatever or whoever is interrupting you can wait until you are finished.

SLEEP

The inability of Alzheimer's patients to sleep at night can be very difficult to resolve. They are frequently sleepier during the day than at night when their sleep patterns tend to be fragmented and disrupted. Some nap off and on both day and night with every hour having periods of wakefulness and light sleep. Such naps help replace the deep, restorative sleep we all need—but it's a major problem for the caregiver, causing serious sleep deprivation. In addition to the disease's inherent sleep problems, there may be pain or discomfort the patient is unable to tell you about. Be alert for urinary tract infections, sleep apnea, restless legs syndrome and depression. The doctor may be able to treat any such conditions.

Sleep medications are not always effective and sometimes make the patient more agitated. Such medications in the elderly, especially with existing cognitive impairment, can be risky. They may result in more falls and fractures, increased confusion, and some decline in the ability to care for oneself. So the caregiver has to be extra alert. However, there are several sleep medications used in the treatment of insomnia and nighttime behavioral disturbances in Alzheimer's patients and it's worth a discussion with the doctor to try them.

Emphasizing again, most important is that the caregiver does not become sleep deprived—that's the way prisoners are sometimes tortured—it's no joke—your health and caregiving ability will suffer. When nothing else works, family members often take turns at night sleeping outside the patient's room while the other caregiver gets some critical rest, or a night attendant has to be hired. Caregivers must get enough sleep, that's paramount.

Obvious things to avoid are excessive fluid intake before bedtime; no exciting or frightening television, and no television if the patient awakens during the night, soft music if that helps; avoid alcohol, caffeine and nicotine; do not give drugs that have a stimulating effect within several hours before bedtime, talk to the pharmacist about the best dosage time for sleeping for all drugs; in as much as possible, maintain regular bedtime and waking time; maintain regular meal times; try to get in some daily exercise, but again, not during the hours close to bedtime; reduce daytime naps if that works, and although it seems paradoxical, sometimes a nap is good so that the patient does not become too tired to sleep at night. Try the old standbys of milk, extra pillows, maybe a nightlight—otherwise keep the room dark and the house quiet. Draw curtains so that window reflections do not startle the patient, cover or remove mirrors, close closet doors, try to eliminate spooky shadows, and as with children, make a bathroom run. Check room temperature and that bedding, pj's and gowns are comfortable and warm or cool enough.

Do not be surprised if your loved one will not stay in bed alone. They become frightened and feel abandoned when they cannot see their caregiver. I would crawl into bed with my husband, have soft music on, hold his hand or hug him until he fell asleep, then I could get up and do something I wanted to do—and often enough, he'd be just a few steps behind me when I left! If your loved one tends to roll off the bed, lower it as far as possible, put a mat next to it and if he continues to sleep after rolling off, give him a blanket, a pillow and let him stay there for the night, or just keep the mattress on the floor. Some people use guard rails, but there's possible danger if a person tries to climb over, so again, use a mat.

Light, especially morning sunlight, has a lot to do with normal sleep cycles, waking with the dawn, retiring when it gets dark—get as much in your routine as you can. Take your loved one outside whenever possible, and let the sunshine inside.

Some people are just night owls, but for most, things that disturb sleep patterns are jet lag, working nights, spending all day inside with no windows, winter or seasonal blues, daylight savings time changes, changes in body chemistry, and damage to brain cells in diseases like Alzheimer's. Bright light, including certain artificial ones, can sometimes help improve sleep, mental functioning and make people more alert. If you don't have a computer, get your grandchild to do some research on Alzheimer's and 'bright light therapy' or 'full spectrum light.' Call the Alzheimer's Association and consult with your doctor, they should know a thing or two about it. Let there be light!

RESPITE

The most serious mistake that the overwhelming majority of Alzheimer's caregivers make is not paying attention to their own well-being—everything revolves around the loved one's demanding care. Who has time for regular check-ups, seeing a doctor about your own medical problems, the dentist, a mammogram, prostate screening, colonoscopy? It's too hard to get anyone to stay with Mom, they won't know what to do when she _____ (fill in the blank). You'll be gone too long, she'll panic. Caregivers don't eat right, get little exercise, are routinely sleep deprived. They're too busy driving Mom around, feeding, bathing, entertaining, running the house, doing laundry, shopping. This was my own personal history. I always told people I was OK, taking care of myself, but I really wasn't. I neglected my own well-being, even though from time to time I did hire someone in the house for a few hours.

Don't become one of these statistics: 43% of Alzheimer's caregivers fall into a clinical depression that can linger for years, even after the loved one dies; 15% will die before their contemporaries and many will die before the patient they care for; elderly caregivers with a chronic illness have a 63% higher mortality rate then their non-caregiving peers; spousal caregivers suffer three times the depression of others in their age group; half of caregivers spend 46 hours a week caring for a loved one and are on call 24 hours a day, seven days a week—there are no days off, no eight-hour shifts. ***This is in violation of all employment directives—private, government, unions***—take care of yourself first!

Caregivers need respite, that is, temporary relief from their caregiving chores. Most will tell you that they daydream about running away, having some 'me' time alone, but it's not always easy to come by. My husband and son often worked together and he clearly saw his father's changing, having problems doing the things he'd always done before. So, he understood the situation and was available sometimes when I felt overwhelmed. A couple of times I asked him to spend a weekend at home with his Dad so I could get away. But I know not everyone has this option.

I also gave respite to myself. At night, when my husband was asleep, I might take a long bath, watch something special on TV, read or do needlework. My thoughts drifted away from his care completely when I followed patterns, chose threads and watched color stitches form designs. Your interests will be different, but grab a short period of time for yourself whenever you can.

Adult day care is good for both you and your loved one. Many patients say they don't want to go, but if you follow the advice of staff, chances are it will work out. Many offer low costs for those who need it. In most areas of the country, there are vans for the handicapped that will take someone to and from day care for a small fee. It's cheaper than using your own car and much easier on you—you have enough to do. During these few hours you can shop, go to a movie, bowl, take a class, whatever—even nap—such respite time for you is priceless.

Then there are some residential care facilities that will take someone for a few days, and again, patients almost always adjust. Caregivers themselves are often the problem, they cannot tear themselves away from their having to 'do-it-myself' caregiving. Don't feel so guilty! You are not the only one who can do the job, and if something bad happens, it will happen, but chances are nothing will. When you can manage to get away, don't—don't—don't call to see how your loved one is doing. You might feel better if you leave written instructions. Do not expect improvements when you return, it will be back to the same old grind, but with a refreshed attitude. It really helps and don't feel guilty—did I say that? Don't feel guilty!

Call Alzheimer's and other caregiver organizations, senior centers, your church, County or State Departments of Aging, friends and family. When someone trustworthy says, "What can I do to help?" ask if they will commit to stay with your loved one on a specific afternoon every six weeks or so. That's not much and you're worth it.

MEMORY LOSS - AGING OR ALZHEIMER'S?

Think back to your childhood and chances are there were times when you forgot to carry your lunch to school, forgot to do your homework or forgot to brush your teeth. People forget—that's normal. For most, it's all acceptable until they begin to reach middle age, then forget something and—*aghwaaaah,* panic attack, panic attack, *I forgot a word, I'm getting Alzheimer's!* Statistics say you are not—until you start pushing 85 when you've got pretty good odds of about 50-50, and anyway, something else may likely get you first. If such forgetfulness does not interfere with taking care of your daily needs, it just means you need a little more time to remember, like needing more time to walk across the street. Forgetting a word for a bit, remembering it later, is only a little 'hiccup' in your memory—it happens.

Our brains have billions of nerve cells. Unless you have done something self-destructive to kill your own brain cells faster, like excessive alcohol or drug use, few die over a lifetime, but they do shrink. Such shrinkage may partially explain why mental functioning slows as we age. However, serious memory loss can occur when whole clusters of cells are destroyed by something like Alzheimer's. Both situations may cause minutely similar memory loss, but they are two completely different things. Forgetting because of shrinkage is annoying but wholly benign. It may progress somewhat, but it's a world away from the unrelenting progression of Alzheimer's.

Around middle age, we begin to produce smaller quantities of the chemicals we need to relay messages between cells. And, between ages 30 to 70, brain blood flow reduces 15-20%, bringing less oxygen. Maybe the shrinking tissues require less blood, or does less blood cause the shrinkage? Either way, it's normal, not a disease and not to worry.

Attitudes also play a part. In research, elderly Chinese performed as well as their younger counterparts and were less forgetful than older Americans who had the preconceived idea that aging causes an inevitable decline in memory. The implication being that if you expect your memory to worsen, you may be less inclined to try to remember.

Research also indicates that the mental process to remember something new is the same as that needed to retrieve something from long ago. Most elderly remember distant events quite well. Maybe their inability to recall new things is because they don't think it's all that important, they just don't pay close attention. If you don't stay active, have an interest in different things, then why bother to remember something new? Although if you feel all you want to do in your golden years is to watch the grass grow—well, that's OK, too.

But there are stark differences between memory loss with aging and that due to Alzheimer's. If you forgot the name of someone you just met yesterday, that's normal, but if you can't remember who your wife is, that's serious. If you forget to set your alarm for the right time, that's normal, but when you can't remember how to operate the clock to set the alarm, something you've done daily for years, then that's serious. If you forget the exact balance in your checkbook, that's normal, but if you forget how to make change or figure out the tip, that's serious. If you forget where you parked your car at the mall, that's normal, but if you are driving and find yourself in a strange neighborhood with no idea of how you got there and don't know which direction is home, then it's past time to see a doctor.

Besides aging, memory loss can be from depression, side effects of medications, stroke, insufficient vitamins, emotional stress, anxiety, lack of sleep, dehydration, maybe an undiagnosed concussion after a fall—lots of common things. It is not unusual for some older people to become momentarily confused, maybe need a helping hand, but if they do not have difficulty performing familiar tasks, do not have serious language problems, if they are not putting shoes in the microwave, or wandering naked outside in the snow, chances are that forgetting a word now and then is just not something to be concerned about.

GETTING A DIAGNOSIS

Lots of luck getting a straightforward diagnosis when there is a memory problem. Even if told it is Alzheimer's, two years later it might all change to something else like Lewy body disease or frontotemporal dementia. Further, other illnesses and certain life-styles, like excessive alcohol, may be contributing factors to memory loss.

Because there are any number of reasons someone has memory loss, in addition to your regular doctor you might also consider a **geriatrician;** or a **neurologist** specializing in brain disorders; or a **psychiatrist** specializing in mood disorders and how the brain works; or a **psychologist** with specialized training in testing memory, problem solving, language and other mental functions. Don't think you will need or want to see any or all of them! If needed, your doctor can help sort them out.

No matter which doctors are seen, someone should go into the exam room with memory loss patients to understand what is happening. If that is not possible, arrange to speak to the doctor about the exam afterwards because such patients will forget what was told to them before they walk out of the office. You cannot rely on what they tell you about the visit.

There is no exact test that proves someone has Alzheimer's. A medical workup will determine overall health and might identify something else that may be causing memory problems. It's a matter of elimination. If nothing else is found to be causing memory loss, it may be a diagnosis of 'probable' Alzheimer's that is 85-90% effective but only 100% verifiable at autopsy.

The doctor will ask what symptoms the patient has been having, so consider starting a journal when an awareness of memory loss begins. It will help him understand when symptoms began, when they happen and if they've gotten worse. He will evaluate the person's sense of well-being, look for depression, other mood disorders, loss of interest in life and any symptoms that can come with dementia. He'll ask about diet and nutrition; check blood pressure, temperature and pulse; listen to heart and lungs; and collect samples of blood and urine. A neurological exam to assess the functioning of the brain and nervous system may identify a brain disorder other than Alzheimer's, so he'll test reflexes, coordination, balance, muscle tone, strength, eye movement, speech and sensation. A brain scan may be called for.

He will interview family members because the patient may not be fully aware of what is happening. Unconscious adjustments are often made by others to adapt to the patient. Asking a spouse or adult child if they feel uneasy leaving the patient alone helps the doctor get an idea of how intimate relationships may have been subtly changing. The doctor will want to know of any medical conditions that affect other family members, especially if someone may have had Alzheimer's or a related disorder. Take the containers of all prescriptions and over-the-counter medicines plus any vitamins or supplements so the doctor can read dosages and look for interactions or side effects. Have all questions written down so you won't forget anything.

A mini-mental state exam (MMSE) will give the doctor an idea of whether or not the patient is aware of symptoms and will be asked what year, season, date and day of the week it is; count backwards from 100 by 7's; spell 'world' backwards. He will be asked to remember three simple things like a car, a tree and a book. Then the doctor will chat for a bit and ask the patient to name the three items. He may also be shown and asked to name a few things in the office like a pen, a clock, a phone. He could be asked if he knows where the doctor's office is, to complete a common phrase and copy a picture of two interlocking shapes or draw a clock showing the 12 numbers in the right places. There will likely be a three-part instruction, such as: take a paper in your right hand, fold it in half, and put it on the floor.

The MMSE is judged on 30 points. A score of 30 is no dementia; 20-24 is mild dementia; 13-20 is moderate; and less than 12 indicates severe dementia. On average the MMSE score with Alzheimer's patients declines about 2-4 points a year.

It is frustrating but important to realize that medical science is not perfect. **Missing clues** and **misdiagnosing** Alzheimer's and other memory problems is not uncommon. Most doctors try their best, but sometimes it may be 'by guess and by golly.' If you feel yours is not doing everything possible, don't hesitate to go elsewhere.

FALLING

Age is the primary risk factor in falling; and age is the primary risk factor for Alzheimer's—not a happy confluence! One in every three seniors over 65 will fall. Most are not serious, people get up, dust themselves off and keep on going, but falls are the leading cause of fatal and nonfatal injuries in older people.

Those who fall the most are older women—especially Caucasians and Asians (maybe it's the shoes they choose to wear!); seniors unable to stand on one leg for more than five seconds; users of multiple prescriptions and over-the-counter drugs; and elderly people who live alone. Falls are not a natural occurrence with age, and while they cannot all be prevented, many can be avoided.

For **both males and females**—how are your bones and those of your loved one? Have a bone scan to check for osteoporosis. Get enough calcium, eat right, do some osteo-bone-strengthening exercises, and ask the doctor about current osteo-medications? You are less likely to sustain a serious fracture if your bones are strong.

Other **risk factors** include hearing and vision problems, mental confusion and decreased feeling in feet; medications that reduce perceptions or cause dizziness; conditions such as arthritis and osteoporosis; forgetting about household hazards and having unrealistic expectations about current abilities; prior falls leading to 'fear of falling' which causes decreased mobility, stiffness and more falls; weak muscles and joints that won't fully bend will interfere with balance; vertigo; decreased reaction time; leaning on unstable furniture, poor lighting, no handrails on stairs, no grab bars; scatter rugs, plush carpet, uneven surfaces; alcohol use and perhaps an undetected infection and pain; shoes with slippery soles, rubber bottoms, heels higher than 1-1/2 inches; poorly maintained equipment, wheelchairs and walkers must be sturdy and in locked position before getting in and out.

Decrease risk by removing rugs, furniture on wheels, clean up clutter, watch for toys and exposed electrical cords, get bells for pets; wear shoes with good non-slip soles, avoid too much cushioning which alters perception, keep laces tied, nothing flippy-floppy or backless; install sturdy well-anchored grab bars and handrails wherever needed and adjusted to the proper height for the patient; keep walking aids close to bed; maintain proper flooring, no slippery waxing; repair holes or seams in carpet, make sure edges and corners are secure; have pharmacist review all drugs for interactions; eliminate too much glare or shadows with lighting, use night lights, keep stairways well-lit, use higher-wattage bulbs; wipe up spills; store frequently used items at a convenient lower level; limit alcohol; rise slowing after sleeping, lying down or sitting; put non-skid appliqués on floor of showers and tubs, use more grab bars, get a shower seat and raised toilet seat; use handheld shower head on a flexible hose; have non-skid rugs in bathroom. Purchase a personal alarm to wear.

When your loved one falls, remember your back! If he's not bleeding or unconscious, he's OK for the moment. Calm down yourself and give him time to 'collect' himself, five minutes or so. Speak gently, directly into the patient's face, don't fuss or discuss blame. Feel limbs for broken bones and question for pain. If there seems to be any problem cover him with a blanket but, otherwise, don't move him in any way. Do not try to lift him yourself. Remember it takes two strong well-trained emergency workers to pick someone up without injury to themselves.

If you don't need to call 9-1-1, bring a stable chair (maybe from the kitchen) to him. Get him into a crawling position then, using both his hands, have him hold onto the seat of the chair. Slowly help him rise, bending the stronger knee while the other, if necessary, is on the floor for balance. Once up, slowly guide him to sit. If this is too hard for either of you, call for help. Call the patient's doctor to report falls. Aging bones are often brittle and tiny fractures from a fall can cause problems, get them x-rayed, don't just wait and see.

Call 9-1-1 if your loved one reports dizziness, begins to slur words, becomes nauseated, unconscious or bleeding a lot. Check pupils to ensure they are both normal size, if one is unusually larger or smaller, have him transported to emergency.

Sometimes, if he's not hurt, you can sit on the floor next to him and after those few calming minutes, you can say, 'guess we should get up now,' and often enough he will get up automatically. Maybe it's the shock and fear of the fall that has, temporarily, intensified his confusion.

EATING

You sweet talk him, offer a spoonful of yummy food, cajole him to please open his mouth, and instead he turns away, clamps his teeth tighter and might swing a fist at you. Or maybe food is stored in his cheeks because he has forgotten how to chew and swallow. It's hard to believe that he is not being deliberately difficult just to annoy you—but he's not—he has advanced Alzheimer's.

You have to be patient to make the eating process easier for both of you. Try to keep calm, unhurried, allowing yourself plenty of time. Eliminate distractions; turn off the television and radio, have others take their conversations outside. If a loved one is too agitated to eat, stop and try again later. Stress can upset the digestive system for both of you.

As Alzheimer's progresses, eating habits and tastes change so accept that things cannot be what they used to be or what you want them to be. To maintain his dignity, try not to fuss about it and allow your loved one to participate as much as possible in eating by himself, even when it gets messy.

Finger foods allow people to choose what they want and maybe walk around—they won't always sit still for meals. Give them time to look at the food and eat at their own pace. But don't offer too many things at once; making a decision can cause anxiety for someone with Alzheimer's. Try a variety of buttered breads, rolls or muffins, crackers with soft cheese, and waffles. Meats should be moist—chicken, hamburgers, hotdogs, meatloaf, fish fingers or crab cakes, slices of pork, veggie sausages, pizza, hard-boiled eggs quartered, cheese cubes or melted cheese on toast—all sliced in easy to eat pieces. Lots of fruit—sliced apples, pears, apricots, peaches, nectarines, and of course, bananas, melon, pineapple chunks, orange segments, berries, seedless grapes, dried fruits.

Veggies can be raw, steamed, boiled—broccoli and cauliflower florets, carrots, cucumbers, celery, green peppers or parsnip sticks, Brussels sprouts, tomatoes and mushrooms. Bake, roast or boil potatoes, with or without skin, and sweet potatoes. Don't forget favorite sandwiches cut into wedges. Everything can also be left out for snacks.

It is not uncommon for Alzheimer's patients to lose weight, even when eating well. Mostly it is the disease, but there could also be things like depression, sore gums, denture problems, lack of exercise, constipation. Check with the doctor and dentist for help with these problems. Because of damage to the brain, they may no longer understand food is to be eaten—even when they are hungry—so you need to remind them to eat and guide food to the mouth. If they don't want to eat, ask the doctor for an appetite stimulant, but some stop eating altogether and that's that.

Don't have elaborate meals; don't 'set' the table. Remove everything except an unpatterned dish, a soup bowl is best, and a spoon. Keep portions small. Serve fluids in a child's 'sippy' cup; soup in a mug. Sometimes they lose the ability to judge temperature, so you'll have to check that. Small, frequent meals instead of three-squares often works. They may eat new things and often go for sweets—offer pudding, ice cream, pie fillings, nutritional supplements. Give lots of liquids, hopefully several cups each day. If they can use a straw, let them. As time goes on, liquids may need to be thickened for safer swallowing. Thickening products are in the market. As well as water, try fruit juice, gelatin, sherbet—whatever liquids they'll take. You may have to begin to puree foods or try baby foods.

If someone doesn't start to eat, offer the first bite to 'prime the pump' or a small taste on the lips often works. Putting food in front of them without comment and walking away can trigger an automatic response to begin eating. Put one food at a time on a plate with contrasting color: chicken or mashed potatoes on a blue plate—not white.

Never offer food to someone who is drowsy or lying down or leave your loved one alone while eating because of the chance of choking. It is easier to feed someone who is reclining, if you use a long-handled spoon, like those for iced tea or an ice cream soda. If your loved one tends to choke while eating, contact a speech and swallow therapist to learn about eating safely. It's dangerous to squirt liquids into someone's mouth—don't do it!

Some patients have ravenous appetites and seem to eat constantly. They don't realize that they just ate or what they are eating, and obviously this presents a much different challenge.

MYTHS

Few people know all the accurate facts about Alzheimer's disease. I certainly didn't before my husband got it—still don't. While the following is essentially correct, understand that on-going Alzheimer's research will likely change many things. The myths themselves are conflicting. Most people will continue to believe what they choose.

Only old people get Alzheimer's.—While 90% of cases occur in people over 65, it can happen to much younger people in their 30's, 40's or 50's. The youngest that I personally know of is 29.

Men are more likely to develop Alzheimer's than women.—Both sexes get it, but women, who live longer than men, are more likely to develop it as they age. People are living longer so the risk of getting Alzheimer's increases for everyone.

Memory loss means someone is getting Alzheimer's.—No, no, no and again no!! We all forget things on occasion—that's normal. But if you remember later that you forgot, then you were just momentarily distracted, you did NOT really forget. Non-Alzheimer's causes of memory loss can be medication, depression, alcohol, poor nutrition, thyroid, head injury, tumors, stroke, heart or lung disease, infection, delirium, fever, dehydration, dementia and whatever. These conditions can easily cause confusion and odd behaviors, but that doesn't mean Alzheimer's.

Memory loss is part of aging.—Many things—other than age—can contribute to memory loss, but it is not part of normal aging. Senility is too often diagnosed, especially by family, for a range of symptoms that can obscure the real problem. There could be a severe undiagnosed medical condition, impaired hearing and vision as well as causes mentioned above.

No one in my family has ever had Alzheimer's, so I'm not at risk.—No one in my husband's family had Alzheimer's. In some families there is an hereditary factor, but the vast majority of cases are termed *sporadic Alzheimer's*, that is there is no family history, no known cause. My own belief is that it is a recessive gene and it is likely that something happens in someone's life to trigger its outbreak.

Someone in my family has Alzheimer's, so I'm going to get it, too.—Hardly. Statistics say you will not. There may be a slight increased chance that you might, if you are in a family where some members have specific genes that can lead to what is termed *familial Alzheimer's*, but that is no guarantee you will get it. Remember you have genes from many family branches, not just the one member who has Alzheimer's.

Family members are the best caregivers for someone with Alzheimer's.—Sometimes, but it often takes professionally trained people to do it well. Family caregivers grow old and have their own medical problems. When possible, professional caregivers in the home or placement in a good Alzheimer's facility can be best for everyone—including the patient.

Alzheimer's can be cured.—As of today, there is no known medically proven cure, although many claim that there is. Some drugs can help some patients with memory loss and slowing the progress of the disease, but nothing can prevent or cure it.

Embryonic stem cells will cure Alzheimer's.—In the future it may be possible to replace dead brain cells, but such cells from a foreign entity will not restore someone's erased memories.

People with Alzheimer's can still work, they often pretend they don't understand, that they can't do something, look for sympathy, and like to annoy others.—It's tempting to believe that when they act so normal on occasion, but almost always, what you see is what you get.

Alzheimer's is not fatal.—People think you cannot die because you forget the names of your grandchildren, but Alzheimer's is far more than the normal forgetting we all experience. The destruction of cells starts in the areas that control memory. That's how we see it in the beginning, but as it spreads, it destroys the cells that also control our unconscious functions, i.e., heart beat, swallowing saliva, circulation, digestion, elimination, breathing, etc. That's how my husband died, his automatic breathing stopped. Ironically, he was, otherwise, in excellent health.

Alzheimer's is a death sentence.—Alzheimer's is normally a very slow moving disease. With treatment and the help of loved ones, most people learn to live quite normal lives for many years, even decades, enjoying life as much as anyone. That was our experience.

Mercury dental fillings, aluminum cookware, aspartame, fluoride, electrical wires, flu shots and such increase the chance of getting Alzheimer's.—Alzheimer's has been around for centuries when people did not have fillings, get flu shots, nor drink from aluminum cans, so it is unlikely that something in our modern society is causing it.

Things like folic acid, vitamin B, caffeine, curry, garlic, lemon balm, ginkgo biloba, ginseng, aspirin, vegetarianism, and hormone replacement therapy may prevent or have a beneficial effect on Alzheimer's.—Such things have been researched, but so far there's no scientific proof that any of them are effective.

If an Alzheimer's patient doesn't get lost or someone is with him, it's OK to drive.—Never, never. We all get lost on occasion, that's not the problem. It's impaired judgment, changes in vision that have nothing to do with eyeglasses, confusing the gas pedal with the brake pedal, misjudging distance and speed, unable to read traffic signs, and much more.

Alzheimer's is a mental disease.—No way! Many symptoms can be the same, but Alzheimer's is a degenerative medical condition, not a psychiatric disorder.

Alzheimer's patients become violent and aggressive.—Some do, but certainly not all.

Those with Alzheimer's cannot understand what is going on around them.—Most caregivers believe that their loved ones <u>do</u> understand more than they appear to. I came to feel that way about my husband.

A healthy life style with regular exercise, eating right, continuing mental stimulation and advanced education will stave off Alzheimer's.—It couldn't hurt!

If you are comfortable using or not using anything, doing or not doing anything and if you have checked with your doctor, then absolutely continue to do so. Sometimes things just work. Everything doesn't have to have a scientific explanation.

WANDERING

One of the most common dangers for someone with Alzheimer's is the tendency to wander and get lost. Over 60% of those with dementia will wander off at some point, and it is especially stressful for the caregivers and family. Most wandering is done on foot; but if a car is available they can take off and disappear in another city. Even if keys are hidden, at least have a tracking device on any car that may be driven by the patient. They can take off on a bike, a motorcycle, even a horse, who knows!

Like almost everything else with Alzheimer's, why some wander and pace can have a variety of reasons. Sometimes it is just aimless movement, or like my husband, it was a continuation of having always been moving, especially at work. It is unreasonable to expect someone to sit or lie in bed all day. The physical need to move is not only common, but with Alzheimer's it can help keep the patient independently mobile for a longer period of time.

If a person has recently been moved or is going to a new day care or respite program, they may feel lost and set out looking for 'home.' They might start looking for a specific place, person or activity and then forget why they are going and become lost. If they can't see their primary caregiver, they can go out looking for them, so it's always a good idea to let your loved one know you are close by.

Often enough, dementia patients are bored. Being occupied brings a sense of purpose for all of us. Try to keep the person mentally and physically active through games or involvement in daily chores—even if they don't do it right. They often have a lot of excess energy, so maybe walk to a store instead of driving, use stairs rather than an elevator, try gardening or other vigorous activity if that is possible.

Sometimes we walk when there is pain, trying to get away from it. Check with the doctor to see if there is undiagnosed pain, especially a urinary tract infection, or if it may be a side effect of medication, although sometimes certain medications can diminish the need to pace. It might be obvious anxiety, fear, loneliness, isolation, or a response to an hallucination. Talk to your loved ones about such things with reassurance that you will always be there and keep them safe. Or they could be hungry, looking for something to eat, or a bathroom to use. Some tend to wander at the same time, maybe when they always left for work, so try to plan an activity for that time to distract them.

If they seem to be searching for something or someone from the past, ask about it, talk to them and take their feelings seriously. Look at some old photos. Don't dismiss such things as over and done with. They often have a job or task they feel a need to finish, taking care of a small child or getting to work. You can have a work area with projects, papers to shuffle or whatever they were used to doing—and dolls or stuffed toys to care for.

If they have a strong need to keep moving, many men just do, don't hesitate to hire someone to walk with your loved one if you cannot do it yourself, although the exercise will be beneficial to all.

As weather changes and it's dark early at night as well as in the morning, someone with dementia becomes confused and at 2:00 a.m. is ready to get dressed and go to work. Or they just get up and walk around the house. In the morning I'd find my husband had moved the clothes hamper, put his shaver in his shoe, figurines and other small items were here and there, out of place. He was very busy.

It is impossible to have a completely risk-free environment. Because Alzheimer's patients rarely look up, install locks as high as possible on outside doors, gates and windows. Sometimes more than one lock in place works best. Make certain that other family members know how to quickly open a locked door in case of an emergency. Matches and other dangerous items can be removed along with scatter rugs and exposed electric wires.

Be sure your loved one has some sort of identification in case of getting out. Get an identification bracelet from a safe return program. Label clothing with your phone number and address. Have identity cards in wallets, purses or pockets. If you can't find someone right away, don't hesitate to call the local police. Have a recent photo available for them to identify your loved one. Don't scold when they get back. Reassure and love them even more, they may be frightened. Often enough this phase will pass.

FEEDING TUBES

"But we can't just let him starve," families cry, "we have to do something." And that 'something' usually means they want a feeding tube. Nutrition is important for those recovering from an illness and regaining their health. Food, liquids, additional calories along with vitamins and supplements are necessary. But it is different with a terminal illness and although many choose to deny it, Alzheimer's is a terminal disease.

Much of the modern world has come to a curious conclusion about death. It is not to be talked about (as if keeping silent will stave off the inevitable). Wills are not to be written; medical directives are not to be made—leaving survivors with difficult emotional and financial decisions—death is often thought of as a medical failure! To paraphrase the reality, it has been said that a dying man needs to die and there comes a time when it is useless to resist. Not that knowing all of this will make things any easier—most seniors have been through losing loved ones too many times and it always hurts anew.

Only a hundred years ago when people were terminally ill or had a catastrophic accident, everyone knew it was only a matter of time until they died. It was tragic then as it is now, but there was a mournful acceptance, not all this 'life at any cost' activity and frequently against the patient's wishes.

A 2003 study in Oregon involved 102 elderly patients without dementia who voluntarily refused food and liquids. Nurses reported that 94 experienced passing with little pain and suffering. Withholding nourishment at the end isn't starvation as we normally think it is. Studies indicate that without artificial feeding, the body's production of its own endorphins—our natural pain-relieving hormones—makes the patient more comfortable and experience less pain. It's Nature's way of a peaceful passing. Why interfere to only make things worse and more drawn out?

Which brings us to feeding tubes and end-of-life decisions. Dying Alzheimer's patients do not recover and get better. Normally they lose their appetite and drop weight. A forced feeding regime can be counterproductive, ineffective. There is no evidence that it will help pressure sores, reverse weight loss or bring beneficial nourishment, prevent aspiration pneumonia, provide comfort, improve any function or extend life past a few days or weeks. Further, it can cause physical pain and emotional trauma for the patient and those who love him. Complications like diarrhea, tube leakage, gastro problems, infections and possibly the use of restraints if the patient is pulling at the tube can occur. In Alzheimer's, the brain is shutting down the body's functions, including digestion and elimination. To force food into a body unable to process it will only cause more problems.

Well, what to do! What to do! The alternative is hand feeding. It may not prevent malnutrition and dehydration, but it gives the patient comfort and intimate care. The caregiver feels useful—doing something caring and loving. Staff in facilities don't have time to hand feed all their patients, but families can come in and do so. Feeding someone can be a very emotional activity and it is easy to conclude that a patient not getting nourishment is being neglected—not having good care. Caregivers have a hard time doing nothing, they feel helpless—and often they are.

But there are still things to do, care to give, love and affection to share without forcing food into a body shutting down. Comfort things can and should still be done. A dry mouth can be relieved with wet mouth swabs, ice chips, products to soothe chapped lips. Keep the mouth fresh by gently brushing teeth—plain water will do. Don't expect your loved one to spit out toothpaste or mouthwash.

Offer a little ice cream, gelatin, candy. Junk food and fast food are OK. Eating only a bite or two is for momentary enjoyment, not nutrition. And always offer favorite home cooked specialties. Try not to nag: "Please, Mom, just take one spoonful of this soup I made just for you." Don't show annoyance.

Absolutely consult with your physician, find out all the pros and cons about feeding tubes so that you can make an informed decision. Each case, each family is different. If others are involved, have a meeting to discuss it thoroughly. They can talk to their own doctors, have their own opinions, get the facts, thrash it out, but always respect the wishes of the loved one—that's paramount.

Remember there are two different groups of patients: One is expected to get well, their internal organs are not shutting down and a feeding tube can bring a positive improvement; the others are terminal, it's a completely different situation.

DRIVING - (PART 1 OF 2)

For a long time I sat in the passenger seat noticing that my husband's driving habits were changing. He drove slower, didn't follow as close to other cars, avoided the freeways, frequently asked me directions—and I had no thought that anything was wrong—that he had become a dangerous driver. Along the way, he'd been diagnosed with 'short-term memory loss,' and on my own I thought he had dementia, but I never connected any of it to changes in his driving.

As his dementia worsened, we went to another doctor who reported him to the Department of Motor Vehicles (DMV). That's the law in California, doctors have to report drivers with dementia and I'm glad. When his license was replaced with an identification card that looked exactly the same, he knew he could no longer drive and he never challenged that. He still had enough reasoning power that he told me it was a good thing. If he had an accident, even if it wasn't his fault, and they got his medical records—which legally they can—we could be sued for everything we had. He knew all along that something was wrong. I was the dolt.

Some warning signs of unsafe driving problems are: confusing the gas and brake pedal; failing to notice stop signs or signals; loss of confidence while driving; riding the brake; others honking their horns; hitting curbs; scrapes on the car, mailbox or garage; driving too slow; confusion at exits; using a co-pilot; getting lost in familiar places. Other telltale signs of driving safety do not have to happen on the road. If someone is having trouble reading, cooking, getting dressed, using the TV remote or the phone, unable to find things they always found before, trying to repair things in an inappropriate way—and certainly if there has been any decline in any mental tests

54

doctors administer—all these things transfer to the inability of safely operating the car. It usually becomes obvious to the driver and to his family, but what to do about it—what to do? It is not surprising that many try to hide it and don't think it is all that serious.

In the very early stages of Alzheimer's, many people are still safe drivers, but when does that change and they become unsafe? Some caregivers admit that they have allowed someone with dementia to continue driving after they felt it was unsafe! Others overreact in the beginning, blaming the disease when the person may have always been a bad driver, or just out of fear. Caregivers should take the time to observe the loved one while driving; keep a written record of driving behaviors that change. Share what you see with your loved one, other family members and doctors.

It is often easier to raise the subject of driving with your loved one in the early stages and discuss possible plans to stop when it becomes dangerous. Your loved one may agree to plan to give up driving in the future, even sign a paper to that effect, but then back out when it comes right down to it. Try to find an opportunity to talk about dangerous driving before it becomes a problem. Don't wait until there is an accident or ticket when you and the driver may dismiss it as a common thing not related to declining abilities.

It is hard for adult children to tell parents to stop driving and the average spouse doesn't want a confrontation. The person closest to the driver, who has seen the changes, is the best one to do this, although the authority of a doctor sometimes works well. A prescription that says 'Do Not Drive' can carry a lot of weight. The doctor may also say that it's only until the patient gets better—or until he sees how the new medications are working. Then it's not so final and chances are the subject will eventually be forgotten. A good time to talk about driving issues is when there's a license renewal needed, a change in medications or some other specific event like a visit to an attorney or accountant—alert that person beforehand about your concerns. Then it can be brought up as part of the planning and what the financial consequences will be if there is an accident. You have to stay flexible about it all but don't lose your focus.

Family members may disagree about not driving. Disagreements can result when one member is aware of the decline while others, who have not ridden with the person, will not see the problem. It is good to have them experience the same things, drive with the person, get on the same page. It has happened that other family members who do not understand the dangers involved have helped an unsafe driver get another key and keep it hidden from the caregiver. You are lucky if friends and family members are with you on this—enlist such help. But too often someone tells a dangerous driver that it's OK to drive. They really do not understand the dangers. And too often, Mom wants Dad to continue to drive because it's easier, Dad doesn't trust Mom to drive and how can they otherwise do the marketing. And don't be surprised if both conveniently forget the doctor's 'Do Not Drive' prescription. Ask the doctor to send a formal letter about not driving; it is something your loved one can refer to when he forgets. Try to keep it the doctor's fault, not yours.

Get a Handicap Parking Permit for your loved one from your DMV. It will make your life so much easier.

DRIVING - (PART 2 OF 2)

If you are concerned about your loved one's driving, there are senior driving programs that will test someone who is having problems driving and if they pass, they are told they can still drive. You should call your Department of Motor Vehicles (DMV), your auto club, senior center or insurance company to find out if such a test is available in your area. If your loved one shows resistance to taking this test, make something up, maybe say it's for an insurance discount—and hope that works. Sometimes those administering these tests do not realize they should be looking for signs of dementia, not someone's ability to drive. They get passed when they shouldn't. So you want to make sure beforehand that the person giving the test knows what to look for. Over and over and over again, when you know something is wrong, family and friends, others in authority—counselors, doctors, instructors—will say it's OK for your loved one to drive—and undercut you. Watch for such things—sometimes it's all but impossible for you to stand your ground.

Frequent, short conversations about driving with your loved one are better than a one-time long discussion. Try to be direct, specific and calm. Remember, those with dementia have difficulty learning and remembering, so they may not recall a conversation about driving and think it is the first time they've heard it. Do not gang up on the driver, it will only cause rebellion. You might broach the subject with a plan already made about who will do the driving for various things. "Susie will drive you to golf on Wednesdays." "Tom is going to take you to the barber." "I'll take you to the grocery on Fridays." Do not rely on a police officer to stop your loved one from driving. Sometimes they stop an elderly erratic driver, and unless they have been trained better, they may escort them, with a friendly or stern warning, in the direction they think is their home and let them go.

Few of us want to stop driving and all that represents. Some are so stubborn they'll drive to their own funeral before they'd give up the keys. Many older people without dementia can assess their own driving and know when to stop, but it's different for those with Alzheimer's. It isn't just a matter of getting lost—we all get lost. Those without dementia know how they got lost and have a good idea of how to get home. With dementia the driver doesn't know that. There are problems with judgment, multi-tasking, slow reaction time, impaired spatial skills and countless cognitive deficits. They will misread a pending emergency, and signs—or not read them at all—they misjudge distance and speed, get flustered. They have visual problems that have nothing to do with normal eyesight and eyeglasses—and many have hallucinations.

It can be incredibly difficult getting someone who has become a dangerous driver to give it up. If you tell them they are not to drive anymore, take away the keys or the license, they will find a way around it. The easiest thing to do in the beginning is to file down one point of the ignition key. The driver still has the key but it won't work. You can lie and say it's the battery; you'll get it fixed tomorrow, but keep putting it off. 'Lose' the auto club card. In a lucid moment the driver may call to get the car towed or fixed, so alert your garage to the problem—don't let them 'fix' it or get new keys. The car can also be 'stolen' and the police just never find it—get someone to do that for you. You can install a remote starter and keep the control on your key chain so that you can drive, but your loved one can't. Or trade the car for a different vehicle and the driver will often be reluctant to drive.

If you are berated, so be it, don't get defensive, don't argue back. Show compassion and understanding. It is useless to explain, argue and reason most of the time, and it often heightens agitation. People will grieve the loss of driving, become angry, sad and confused. It's normal and some time can be spent letting this grief come out, validate their feelings of loss, agree that you don't like this situation either. Let them talk it out, and assure them that you are always going to be there to help. Often, they simply do not understand that they have a problem. If it doesn't cause too many problems, keep the car around if it makes the driver happy. Be creative, lie if need be, you could be saving lives!

It is important to understand your liability if you are a caregiver for someone who has dementia or Alzheimer's and gets into an accident. Your insurance company could say that you knew about it and did not tell them of the medical diagnosis, and you might be on your own to pay. Further, someone can sue and get unlimited amounts of money that far exceed your insurance coverage; you could lose everything—and really feel bad about the whole thing. Since each state is different and insurance companies all have their own claims policies, you might call your insurance company and see where you stand. If someone's license has been lifted, you may want to remove that person from the policy. There are countless scenarios regarding unsafe driving, but inasmuch as possible, you want to protect yourself financially and emotionally, your loved one and any innocent victims who may get involved.

Get a Handicap Parking Permit for your loved one from your DMV. It will make both of your lives so much easier.

SEXUALITY - (PART 1 OF 2)

Some people may be surprised to hear that sex is a big issue with Alzheimer's, whether caring for a spouse, parent or non-parent, whether the caregiving is in the home or a care facility. Many people, at any age, shun sex for their own personal reasons; medical conditions can prevent sexual activity; and suitable partners may be few and far between; but sex is a basic human condition and often stays with people as they continue to grow older.

If it is accurate that sex originates in the brain, then the damage that Alzheimer's does to the brain can change things dramatically. Alzheimer's is far more than a disease of forgetting. As it progresses, it is definitely a disease of regression and with a loss of inhibitions. Some patients forget appropriate public behavior and undress or fondle themselves. They may use vulgar words and act sexually aggressive toward family members and strangers. It is imperative that the caregiver remember that these behaviors are a symptom of the disease and not a reflection of the person's character. Such behaviors, usually never seen before from the loved one, can greatly upset the caregiver. It is important then to get the support needed to deal with and understand these disturbing actions, even if it means seeing a counselor to cope with uncomfortable feelings.

Retired Supreme Court Justice Sandra Day O'Connor recently let it be publicly known that her Alzheimer's husband has fallen in love with a woman Alzheimer's patient in the care facility where they both live. This is not uncommon and it happened to me. My husband took up with a woman in his facility. They were all over each other. I saw it and what I didn't see, I was

60

told. He did, however, introduce her to everyone as 'My wife, Betty Lee,' and when I went to visit, I didn't think that he really knew what my place was in his life anymore—much less hers. She would bang on the door to his room to be let and when staff told her, 'he's married,' she'd yell, 'no, he's mine.' She went so far as to pull him away from my arm, but what was I to do?

Staff said they would keep them apart, they'd seen it all before many times. But I said leave them alone. They are both demented, they don't understand that they are doing something inappropriate. Besides, if my husband was getting individual affection and attention, I was happy for him. His life was otherwise barren enough. Many asked how I could stand it, wasn't I jealous, maybe I should scratch her eyes out! The hard truth is that the man who walked with this woman hadn't been my husband for many years. Oh, God, yes, I still loved him with all my heart and soul, and in his way, I know he still loved his wife, Betty Lee.

I had long ago learned that Alzheimer's controlled both of us; I would do whatever was necessary to keep our lives as calm and serene as possible. If it wasn't this woman, it would be someone else; he was looking for comfort and affection in a tormented life. How could that be wrong when I was no longer around to offer it? If he couldn't open a window, dress himself, find the bathroom—he certainly didn't know about marriage vows and being faithful. I was also told that at night, my husband would take off all his clothes and walk the halls stark naked! Fortunately, I never had to respond to that!

At this time there was a man who came to visit his wife, another patient, three times a week for conjugal visits. I didn't know the woman, had no idea if she was agreeable or not. Was he satisfying his needs without regard to hers, or was she eager to be with him and enjoyed their time together knowing that she was loved? I found that knowledge a bit unsettling and could never put it into a comfortable context.

But I do know that marital love can easily go from passion to platonic when your spouse has Alzheimer's. The eternal misunderstandings, arguments, frustrations and physical exhaustion of the caregiving spouse will cause intimacy to vanish. And male or female, changing your loved ones diapers will put off the most ardent

Wives complain that their previously sexy husbands have become clumsy, inept, forgetful and don't seem to be 'there' in the moment. Husbands complain that wives have become so childlike that they feel as if they are raping a child. How do you have intimacy with a man who calls you 'Mommy' or a woman playing with dolls? For many caregivers, the love and years of building a life together does not die but keeps them even closer to their spouse as time goes on. They never neglect the care of their mate, but life as a husband or wife as they knew it, the partnership, is forever gone.

Before my husband got Alzheimer's and even afterwards, I met spouses who had on-going relationships with others, and I wondered how they could manage that. I even had people tell me I should start to date again. Not easy to do when every moment was devoted to caring for my husband. I had neither the time nor the energy! I used to call myself a 'married widow,' living in limbo. Once a man showed interest in me, asked if I was married, and I said 'yes, I am.' But inside I was thinking, 'I don't know if I'm married or not anymore, vows and a piece of paper do not a marriage make.'

As with anything in life, we must make our own decisions. In the years I lived with Alzheimer's and have written about it, I think I have heard all the pros the cons, the 'for better or worse,' arguments, 'til death do us part,' etc. But what do you do when the marriage itself has died? And Alzheimer's changes marriage to the point that it is unrecognizable.

Sex, of course, is only one part of life and marriage, but for many, it does loom heavy. It's another case of your having to walk in someone else's moccasins before you fully understand and make a judgment.

SEXUALITY - (PART 2 OF 2)

Thirty year old Susan has been caring for her widower Dad with advancing Alzheimer's for a few years. In recent weeks he has become sexually aggressive toward her, his own daughter, and this upsets Susan to the point that she is thinking of placing him in a care facility.

He grabs her breasts, puckers up to kiss her lips, and talks intimately about their rolling in the hay. "Stop that, Dad, stop that," Susan demands, backing away from his groping. But he continues trying to verbally cajole her into his bed until she flees the room, crying and bewildered. What has happened to her loving, protective father who has never touched her in an inappropriate manner, how did he become a dirty old man engaging in incest and sexual abuse?

Several unseen and misunderstood things are happening. Alzheimer's is a disease of regression and Susan's Dad is slipping back into his thirties. His daughter looks like his wife did at that age; he doesn't realize nor recognize that they are two different women, his wife has died and decades have gone by. His behavior is perfectly normal and acceptable for a young husband. Now he becomes bewildered, why has his playful wife suddenly become so stand-offish? He's understandably angry.

Dad's sexual behavior may very well pass as he moves into another stage, and it is up to Susan to decide if she wants to continue with his care or hire others, although having another young woman as her Dad's caregiver may well continue his actions. But a male or an older professional woman, well-trained and acquainted with the vagaries of Alzheimer's will be understanding and know how to handle things.

In the meantime, once Susan understands what is going on, she can get some control of things if she enters his room with a "Hi, Dad, it's me, Susan," reality-check greeting. Most Alzheimer's patients still crave affection and personal touch, Susan will want to offer that to her Dad, but she has to do it in a way that does not spark intimacy. It helps if she responds to his need for closeness with talk that involves distractions about other family members, reminiscing and favorite activities.

Alzheimer's women often mistake the actions of a male doctor as a sexual advance. They may well respond in kind, or gently reassure the doctor that he's a very nice man, but she's already married to Robert Redford or Clark Gable—and in her current state of mind, she is! A son, caring for Mom, can have the same misunderstood sexual encounters as Susie has with her Dad. Most children, opposite sex or not, do want to take care of their parents.

It's a fine line to be sensitive and reassuring, while being aware of conditions that may provoke sexual interest. Firm limits for behavior must be set, redirect the person to something else or put it off—'we can talk about that tomorrow.' Responding to loneliness with gentle talk, a caring pat or hug, without over responding, can establish a balance between the patient and caregiver. But all this bathing, loving dialogue, care, attention and diaper changing can have unintended consequences for everyone. It may not happen, but if it does, it's just one more problem to cope with in the mix of caregiving for someone with Alzheimer's and you have to give it some intense thought to keep it under control.

Sexual advances are not limited to family, it happens in public and in care facilities, patients making up to staff or each other, seeking affection and affirmation, even fondle themselves or each other. Elderly patients may behave like teen-agers at the mall, flirt, make crude remarks. Try not to overreact or express shock; don't get angry or argue; don't ridicule or shame; gently remind your loved one that their behavior is not appropriate; be sensitive and reassuring; and if in a public place, do not hesitate to apologize and explain to someone that the person you are with has an illness. Most people will understand.

Alzheimer's patients lose their inhibitions due to changes in the brain, not because they have turned nasty on purpose; the brain may suddenly have an insatiable sexual desire that they act on but don't fully understand; there can be misunderstood circumstances that suddenly provoke excessive sexual interest; like mistaking someone for one's partner or forgetfulness.

And then there is the undressing—completely undressing. Sometimes an Alzheimer's patient's skin becomes sensitive, try to keep clothing soft and loose, maybe try a soothing lotion; clothing can be too tight; it can be hot weather or an overheated room; the person may need to use the bathroom; or it could be boredom and undressing is something to do. It is not a sign of sexual exhibitionism; it's a loss of inhibitions in the brain.

Like most of us, people with Alzheimer's often crave love and affection and will find it wherever they can. All of this may make you uncomfortable and challenge many of your life-long beliefs, but it is imperative that you understand it is the disease and not any social or moral defect in your loved one.

PROGRESSION

When getting a diagnosis of Alzheimer's, it is not uncommon for people to wonder about a prognosis and how long it will last. Surprising to many, it can last more than 20 years or as little as two or three. There are countless variables to consider, while at the same time, few absolutes that apply to every case—that's the nature of the disease. Often, the younger the person is at onset, the more rapid the progression, although that is not always true. Similarly, the rate of decline can be faster when there is a strong family history of the disease.

Statistics say that by age 85, half that population will have Alzheimer's and, by then, few can expect a life expectancy of another 20 years. Many will have heart problems, diabetes, cancer or more—any of which can take them before Alzheimer's. The same is true even with much younger people in their 50's or 60's who have other life-threatening diseases, other things can intervene. Even life style may play a part. Those who are more sedentary can develop problems with movement that may lead to falls, less muscle strength, poor circulation, and perhaps experience a shorter course of the illness than others who have been more active. Generally, someone with Alzheimer's will live about 7 years after diagnosis, but remember, people can have the disease for many years before a diagnosis is made, so again, the pace of known progression varies with the individual. Still, Alzheimer's is often very slow moving and it is not unusual for people to have many years of a very good life. My husband certainly did.

Such erratic progress is not confined only to Alzheimer's. It occurs with diseases like cancer that can be incredibly aggressive in one person and somewhat mild in another. For many, treatments are effective and improving all the time, some will live a good long lifetime, others will not. But with Alzheimer's both the mind and the body are involved making it a whole different ballgame to deal with.

Eventually, people involved with Alzheimer's hear about 'stages' and want to know what they are and what stage one is in, how long will the stage last, what changes can be expected, what will happen in the next stage, how long can someone live? These stages are just a way of gauging the progression of the disease in any one individual and they are not absolutes. It is easy to get hung up on the stages, but they are too flexible to apply to each patient in a consistent, helpful way. There are those who want to know everything beforehand, what to look for, and plan how they will cope. They read and question everything, feel more in control. This can be very empowering, but Alzheimer's is often too elusive to always have a handle on it. Then, there are people like me. I was perfectly willing to greet each new day and each new behavior as it occurred. Then—and only then—would I deal with it.

Stages were essentially developed within the Alzheimer's medical community to categorize patients, in a general way, as they change. It helps doctors monitor progression, researchers to compare groups of patients with one another, and the family to have an idea of the overall condition of a loved one. Although they are useful to determine the level of care a patient will need, they are not terribly helpful as a prognostic indicator because of the great variability exhibited by different patients.

Still, knowing the stages can be helpful on the surface if one is thinking about placement, financial planning, continued home caregiving, selling a house, family dynamics and such to have an idea of what is likely to happen within a reasonably expected time frame. Because of my husband's small business, our finances and medical decisions had been taken care of years before Alzheimer's ever entered our lives. It is much easier if you don't have to make such decisions under emotional stress and being up against the wall—and these decisions will have to be made eventually—there's no avoiding them. The longer they are put off, the harder they are to deal with. Whatever level of progression your loved one is in at the moment, if your legalities are not already in place—now—today—then make an appointment and get it done tomorrow.

Progression by stages varies a bit even with experts, but in most scenarios it begins with no overt symptoms of Alzheimer's, or maybe some mild cognitive decline which will be chalked up to stress, age, depression, drinking or just being quirky. Seldom, if ever, does anyone suspect a brain disease, although the patient may feel that something is wrong but not talk about it. Tests are coming on line that will be able to detect Alzheimer's earlier, before any of the bizarre behaviors arise. That's important because as more medications and treatments come out, they can be given sooner and, hopefully, help slow the speed of the progression. But for the most part, it is still well hidden in the first stage of the early years.

STAGES AND THE CAREGIVER

It is sometimes difficult to know which Alzheimer's stage someone is in because each patient is different, symptoms often overlap, some behaviors never occur, and duration times vary. There's a lot of wiggle room and different designations, but the generally accepted Seven Stages of Alzheimer's are shown here, not only on how they affect the patient, but just as important on how they impact the caregiver. Comments for caregivers are presented in (*italics*).

1. **No impairment**—The patient may have problems remembering names and finding the right words but still functions normally. Such memory lapses will often be attributed to aging, stress, depression—and that may be what is going on. It's too soon to know whether or not things will progress to Alzheimer's, it may be something else. Patient appears normal, even to doctors.

    (It is important to see a doctor as soon as even minor cognitive changes are observed. Find out what it is. The sooner it's caught, the better things are likely to be. Most wait too long. Legal, financial and medical planning must be done <u>now</u> before cognitive decline worsens.)

2. **Very mild cognitive decline**—There is short-term memory loss, an inability to learn and retain new information, depression, apathy and refusal to seek treatment. Mood changes occur, anger develops—it's sharp and it's quick, conflicts arise. Frustration will increase, emotions are more intense. Colleagues often notice changes first but chalk it up to problems at home. The patient seems willful and self-absorbed.

(The caregiver is not believed by family and others, will become defensive, lash back and argue, accuse the loved one of being deliberately difficult, doing and saying hurtful things on purpose. Because these changes are not consistent and there will be many perfectly normal times, the caregiver naturally thinks it can all be controlled, but it can't. The caregiver begins to realize the usual way of handling things won't work and reaches out to support groups and Web sites.)

3. **Mild cognitive decline**—Patients have trouble paying bills and managing finances. They cannot make change, figure a tip, or decide what to buy. They have trouble accessing familiar Web sites and understanding written material. They fall prey to TV, phone, mail order and internet scams. They have difficulty taking phone messages and are unable to use familiar tools. Guns become a danger. They become unsafe drivers.

(It is the wise caregiver who quickly makes arrangements to prevent the loved one from accessing any significant amount of money. All guns must be removed from the home—no exceptions. The biggie now is to get them to stop driving. It can cause terrible scenes, but it must be done. Lay the blame on the doctor who will, hopefully, cooperate and notify the authorities.)

4. **Moderate cognitive decline**—Patients obsess and worry about when things will occur. They lose reading comprehension; forget how to use a phone. They don't see things getting dirty, the bathroom is soiled, clutter develops. Cooking skills are lost. Making a sandwich is too confusing. Weight loss may occur. The stove and running water are left on, doors not closed. The house is too hot or too cold, and a loved one may wear a winter coat on a sizzling day. They withdraw from social activities, lose their sense of danger, become more irritable, frustrated,

self-absorbed and unable to plan ahead. They may deny any memory problems and argue about that. They are angry about lost activities, especially driving and may lose any sense of humor. They will not recognize their own house and want to go 'home.'

(The caregiver is also getting more irritable and frustrated, thinking 'what about ME and MY life?' Caregivers learn to stop telling loved one anything in advance. They begin to lie to loved one to avoid arguments and conflicts that have no resolution. Keeping things calm becomes more important than winning a fruitless argument. The house and everything in it becomes a potential danger, caregiver must always be on alert and begins to lock up dangerous items, social life disappears. Caregiver neglects own well-being, missing medical appointments, afraid to leave loved one alone, is feeling trapped.)

5. **Moderately severe cognitive decline**—Self-care declines. There is refusal to bath, fear of water, wanting to wear the same clothes, getting angry about changing clothes or laundering them, or they may change clothes a lot, selecting odd combinations, and need help getting dressed. On occasion they forget family and friends. They cannot understand TV, mirrors, innate objects; have problems with too much noise and stimulation. They repeat and repeat and repeat, lose language ability, become more and more self-centered, unable to reason and make decisions. Clings to caregiver. Pacing, wandering, unable to sleep, late day confusion and 'seeing' others in the house begins.

(Caregiver considers quitting work, getting help at home. TV has to be monitored. Caregiver can't get a minute alone even for a bathroom break, makes decisions without consulting loved one and becomes severely sleep deprived. Continual repeating is hard to take. Hearts are broken when loved one does not recognize family members.)

6. **Severe cognitive decline**—Total loss of bladder and bowel control. Shuffling, trouble sitting down or standing up, feet seem nailed to the floor, falls occur, head hangs forward, there is severe leaning, doesn't know family at all, accuses them of stealing, being imposters, liars, may become aggressive. Has to be coaxed to eat, refuses food with clenched teeth, or has to be spoon-fed, may put non-food items in mouth, picks up imaginary mites. Little language left.

   (Caregiver is completely exhausted physically, mentally and emotionally. Health is suffering, needs respite and that's often hard to get. Conflicted about need to place loved one in a care facility, guilt is overpowering and leads to inertia.)

7. **Very severe cognitive and physical decline**—Moves about aimlessly, dependent on others for everything, forgets to chew and swallow, may choke on thin liquids, aspiration pneumonia is possible, severe weight loss. Sleeps most of the time, urinary tract infections may be frequent, lies motionless in bed or assumes fetal position.

   (It is the rare caregiver who can continue to do it alone. Hospice or placement is required to <u>save the caregiver</u>. If not already done, decisions must be made about end of life choices. A feeding tube? Hospital admission? What to do when caregiving is over? How to get back into the work force, develop new friends, build a life without the loved one?)

   Patients may rally, have brief moments of lucidity or worsen. Medications, other medical conditions, fatigue, too much change or activity all play a part. *(The best the caregiver can ever do is the best that the caregiver can ever do—and the best that the caregiver can ever do is <u>enough</u>.)*

CATEGORIES & GENES

Most people still cling to the belief that Alzheimer's is something that happens to old men when they retire—a gentle, often amusing forgetfulness. Older ladies get pixilated; the elderly naturally get senile, especially if they don't keep mentally and physically active. Isn't that so? Isn't it all just part of life, of aging? Well, no, although one can devoutly wish that it was. What it is, without any qualifications, is a disease of the brain. It is not, absolutely not aging, a mental or psychiatric disorder and, no matter what those close to them may think, people who suffer from Alzheimer's do not do things on purpose to annoy others nor can they help their odd behaviors, even though they will often have moments of normalcy.

Alzheimer's is divided into different categories. The most common and well known is _Late Onset_ or _Sporadic Alzheimer's Disease_ affecting about 90% of sufferers, usually occurs in people over age 65, and appears to affect about 50% of those over age 85. There didn't seem to be a common link among those who got it so researchers have had a difficult time identifying causes. But ongoing studies throughout the world keep finding new clues, it's still very fluid. Just recently, a discovery of a new genetic risk factor has been found. Events like this are critically important. They may lead to new specific medications or, perhaps, find that some existing ones will be beneficial. There may be more to the cause than just one specific gene; maybe there's a family history, the role of heredity is still being studied; and whether someone has a specific gene or not, there is no test to determine if any given person will develop the disease.

Early Onset Alzheimer's Disease (EOAD) happens when people are diagnosed before age 65, usually in their 50's. While rare, it can develop in the 40's, even the 30's. The youngest I personally know of is 29! They also tend to decline faster. Much less than 10% of all cases are this type—maybe less than 5%. Younger people appear to have more of the microscopic changes found in the brain than those with late onset and EOAD has its own genetic defect that is not linked to that of late onset. But the symptoms are the same. Because they are younger, patients may be more physically fit and socially active with careers and young families still to raise. When one has these other issues to deal with daily, caregiving becomes more challenging and will require additional methods and support to cope. In consequence, they might react differently to the disease than the elderly, to feel more cheated, depressed, powerless, frustrated, and pulled in both allegiance and time. Effects on children and grandchildren from all this turmoil in the home can be devastating.

These defective genes are found throughout the human race, but the subsequent appearance of Alzheimer's differs among whites, blacks and other groups, even between Europeans, occurring at 30% in Lapps, Swedes and Finns to 10% to 12% with Greeks, for example. Because of cultural differences, extended families who may share caregiving, reluctance to see a doctor, misdiagnosis, finances, and social taboos, it can be difficult to achieve accurate statistics, but all races appear to get Alzheimer's, one way or another.

Familial Alzheimer's Disease (FAD) is entirely inherited through a pattern where members of at least two generations in a family have had Alzheimer's. If one parent carries the inherited gene, each child has a 50% chance of getting it, but it is not preordained. It is extremely rare, accounting for less than 1% of all cases. It has a much earlier onset, often in the 40's, and can clearly be seen to run in families. However, the presence of more than one family member with Alzheimer's does not necessarily mean it is specifically familial.

(I do not have a scientific background so I cannot discuss details of various research programs about the brain and causes of the disease, I can only relate, through research, the published conclusions of experts in the field. All such research is pretty much in its infancy and often changes with each new discovery. Not every expert agrees with every other one 100% of the time. Differences in statistics, opinions, and conclusions are built into the elusive nature of Alzheimer's. For instance, it is known that some people with the guilty genes get the disease while others who also have the same genes do not and no one, as yet, knows why. Information is all over the Internet and at the library for those who want to learn more. But the who? how? when? and why? of the basics will continue to be probed and studied for some time. We will all learn the advances and the disappointments together.)

So does it really matter who has which kind? It matters to those in the medical research field as they continue to seek causes and, hopefully, prevention, medications and treatments. But, maybe, not so much for the patient, family and caregivers because the bizarre behaviors and the loss of essence of the self are the same. But the family life issues are quite different and no matter the category, it behooves people to look for support from others with like problems.

People are sometimes reluctant to join a support group and often enough, in smaller communities, they may not even exist. Whether caring for a parent or spouse, the relationships change. The adult child becomes the parent, a spouse becomes a parent—someone has to be in charge. Emotional bonds between child and parent are very different from those between spouses. And, these lifelong relationships don't change overnight or with ease. The anxiety, guilt, sadness, physical, emotional and mental responsibilities take their toll. It helps tremendously if you can receive and offer understanding; exchange information and ideas; and talk with others caring for a loved one on the same path. There's a world of difference between a young family going through EOAD and those who are quite elderly, but even if you can't find one of your own level, attend a support group anyway.

The National Institute on Aging has Alzheimer's or memory clinics at major medical institutions, hospitals and universities throughout the country. Call them or your State's Department of Aging to find the one nearest you. And get on a computer. Search for 'Alzheimer's Message Boards,' visit several; communicate with others who will be incredibly helpful. If you can not do it yourself, get your grandkids or other youngsters on it, they'll be happy to show you.

HOSPICE & PALLIATIVE
(COMFORT) CARE

The term 'hospice' (from hospitality) dates from medieval times when it referred to a place where weary travelers stopped for shelter on a long journey. It was first used in modern times by physician Dame Cicely Saunders in 1967 when she founded St. Christopher's Hospice in London, England, the first such facility as we know them today.

Until recent times, life and death were clear cut, there was not all the lingering and intervention we are so dependent on now. If you were gravely ill or had a serious accident, hopefully, you got well. But if you were unable to breathe, you stopped breathing and died, if unable to swallow food, you did, indeed, starve, if bleeding internally, you bled to death. While heartbreaking then, as now, this is Nature's way. Today we fight death to the last second, life at all cost, sometimes causing more harm to the patient than comfort. It's as if society has determined that death is no longer a viable option, not inevitable and far too frightening to face. For many, there is simply no letting go, and, too often, the patient has little say in the matter.

Because of medical advances that we almost all treasure, society is now faced with legal, political, biotechnological, bioethical and religious questions that were never considered before and will, likely, never be fully resolved. And so we have hospice—to ease each other through that bordering limbo between life and death. Do not mistake hospice for doing things that will make the patient better—although, on occasion, that has happened—it is to provide care and comfort for the terminally ill and their families. It is usually in the home, but is also available in many care facilities. In most states it is covered by Medicare, but each state is different. Among other services, in addition to medical palliative (comfort) care, hospice provides physician and nursing services, respite for caregivers, spiritual and bereavement care and counseling.

In palliative care, no specific therapy is excluded for consideration. The individual's needs are constantly assessed and all possible treatments explored and evaluated for bringing comfort to the patient. Family, patients and physicians, together, determine the most suitable care. Hospice teams manage pain and other symptoms; assist the patient with emotional and spiritual aspects of dying; provide drugs, medical supplies and equipment; and deliver certain physical therapies.

Experienced hospice personnel know how to interpret gestures and the often unspoken language of the terminally ill that can bring comfort to both the dying patient and the family. They understand the patient's need to communicate, their requests for a peaceful death, how to respond and recognize their wishes.

It is only in recent years that the medical establishment has come to realize that Alzheimer's patients and their families need hospice and the comfort care it provides as much as others traditionally served. The general public still has a hard time understanding that Alzheimer's is a terminal disease and that the end-stage often brings serious physical problems that demand professional care. The burden on the at-home family caregiver can be far more severe and debilitating than for many other conditions.

Studies have shown that end-stage Alzheimer's patients receive too frequently aggressive treatments, including feeding tubes, with little or no medical benefits. They also receive fewer analgesics (pain relief) then those who are still cognitive. In nursing homes, many receive a regimen of antibiotics, often intravenously, in their last two weeks of life. Yet, research has shown no real difference in survival rates between patients treated and those untreated.

Medical science is learning more and more about Alzheimer's, what will work and what will only prolong the imminent. Why have we resisted offering palliative care for end-stage Alzheimer's for so long? Perhaps because patients are unable to express their pain and needs? But, they, along with all dementia patients, need caring comfort instead of treatments that are frightening, painful and completely ineffective. There comes a time when they just need us to be there with them, to comfort and provide for their wishes. They deserve pain control, companionship, hygiene, physical and emotional contact to know that they still matter. Too often we do not realize that because someone is elderly, demented and unable to speak that their quality of life is underestimated. But palliative care can protect such patients from useless procedures. Professionals can also help the family to more thoroughly understand what is happening to a loved one. Sometimes, the procedures that save the rest of us are harmful to the Alzheimer's patient as the body is shutting down.

Palliative care can be offered any time during an illness. In that way it is different from hospice which is usually relegated to end-stage. Nor is it linked to euthanasia, it does not hasten death nor prolong the dying process. It is Nature taking its course without drastic medical interference—that cannot stop it anyway. Programs have been introduced in the past several years to integrate palliative care into the treatment plans for Alzheimer's patients—good medical practice.

If we accept Alzheimer's as a terminal illness and educate the public, staff in hospitals and nursing homes about palliative care for patients, more and more families will seek such assistance. There should also be discussions with the patient, family and caregivers about preferences when the patient still has the mental capacity to make any wishes known. Someone needs to have durable power of attorney for health care to see that any personal plans and decisions are carefully followed. Finally, just our human presence in the palliative setting for end-stage Alzheimer's patients will maintain their dignity, allay fears and reassure them that they are important and always loved. They deserve no less.

EARLY DETECTION MATTERS

Nobody knows when Alzheimer's really begins, but it is certainly there years before—if not decades before—the bizarre behaviors come raging out and it's apparent that 'something' is terribly wrong. There are documented cases of people in their 20's and I think my husband was one of them—not documented, of course; in the 1950's few even knew what the word 'Alzheimer's' meant.

Ours was a traditional romantic love story; we had every reason to live happily ever after, growing old and fragile, walking hand in hand slowly into the sunset. We traveled married life closely together but each on our own path. He let me be me, I let him be him. If he was quirky and sometimes preoccupied, I knew it was stress, problems at work, whatever. He was always there for me and the kids, life was good. But when others asked 'why did he say *that*?' or 'why did he do *that*?' I'd get annoyed and say, 'why ask me, ask him?' I just didn't see anything wrong. Well, that's not quite true; I'd see fear and terror in his eyes from time to time although he was the bravest man I knew. We all have our little nightmares, but not like what I saw and he would never confide in me. Fifty years later, I know Alzheimer's was always there, I just didn't recognize the warning signs. But he knew 'something' was wrong and was terrified because he was losing his mind. For years I've felt this way alone, most continue to dismiss me.

But a man named Jay Smith knows. Smith says, "It took more than two years for my wife to obtain a correct medical diagnosis, so we decided to do everything we can to increase early detection of Alzheimer's . . . to help others along the way". His wife, Patty, is only 51, which means she obviously had it for some years in her 40's. Smith submitted his *Alzheimer's*

Disease: Early Detection Matters project to American Express. The card company had conducted a campaign to determine which medical project should receive research money. All applicants were worthwhile, but Smith received the most card member votes. The Alzheimer's Association will receive $1.5 million from American Express to implement an *Early Detection* program. Way to go, Smith! And kudos to American Express.

Early detection is critical and incredibly difficult to recognize—even by experts. Such knowledge, years before it is even suspected, will lead to knowing how to live with and understand many of the hidden complexities of the disease and, hopefully—hopefully, slow its progression, if not find a cure or prevention.

Projects in the pipeline may lead to early detection and possible development of pharmaceuticals to slow the onset. Blood test are being worked on that can show a predisposition to Alzheimer's and even distinguish between Parkinson's, Alzheimer's, Lou Gehrig's disease or tell whether a patient is disease free. Blood draws are done with relative ease. There is less discomfort and costly expense than spinal taps, which is typically the way markers may be found in the plasma of early Alzheimer's patients.

Computers are being used to read brain scans to diagnose Alzheimer's faster and more accurately than clinicians. They can distinguish between Alzheimer patient's scans and those with other forms of dementia, such as frontotemporal dementia. Early accurate diagnosis can greatly improve chances of effectively slowing deterioration.

Another early detecting tool is a brain-imaging method that employs radioactive dye injected into the blood stream, it then travels to the brain and attaches to plaque deposits believed to cause Alzheimer's. The dye makes the plaque look yellow on the scan so that it's readily seen.

Even our eyes are being studied. There is an optical test that can determine the presence of the same markers found in the brain of Alzheimer's patients that are in the lens and fluid of their eyes. None of these research projects are 100% positive, only an autopsy is proof positive, and no one knows which will be effective or what others may come along. But it is an indication that the Alzheimer's community is coming to understand that this vicious disease is living with us years before we even suspect its presence.

Ten Warning Signs—What's normal and what's not. Don't panic! Statistics are on your side.

1. Memory loss: Forgetting recently learned information is one early sign. It becomes more frequent and the person is unable to recall the information later. Normal: Occasionally forgetting names or appointments is common, but when you remember them later, it's not Alzheimer's.

2. Difficulty performing familiar tasks: It is hard to plan or complete everyday tasks. People lose track of steps to prepare a meal, use the telephone or play a game. Normal: Occasionally forgetting why you came into a room, where you parked your car, or a word, is *not* Alzheimer's. Stop worrying!

3. Problems with language: Those with Alzheimer's will often substitute different words for a forgotten one. A toothbrush becomes 'that thing for my mouth'. Normal: Sometimes having trouble finding a word is OK. It is estimated there are anywhere from 700,000 to a million words in English, more than any other language. Give yourself a break!

4. Disorientation to time and place: It's easy to become lost in your own neighborhood, forget how you got somewhere and not know how to get home. Normal: Forgetting the day or where you're going on occasion is why we have calendars and a GPS.

5. <u>Poor or decreased judgment:</u> Wearing layered clothing when it's hot or shorts and a tank top when it's cold, giving away money to telemarketers or someone on TV is not good. <u>Normal:</u> Making a questionable or debatable decision from time to time is really embarrassing, but at least we know what we did!

6. <u>Problems with abstract thinking:</u> Those with Alzheimer's have trouble with mental tasks, like not understanding what numbers represent or how they are used. <u>Normal:</u> Finding it challenging to balance a checkbook or do your own taxes. You're competing with computers for goodness sakes.

7. <u>Misplacing things:</u> Someone with Alzheimer's may put a garden hose in the clothes hamper, a cell phone in the microwave. <u>Normal:</u> Misplacing eyeglasses or keys is common. I have at least five pairs of eyeglasses around the house and sometimes I still have trouble finding one.

8. <u>Changes in mood or behavior:</u> Someone with Alzheimer's may show rapid mood changes for no apparent reason—calm to tears to anger. <u>Normal:</u> Nobody's life is always smooth; we all have our moments, but usually know why.

9. <u>Changes in personality:</u> It's common for them to become suspicious, fearful, confused, dependent and cling to the person closest to them. <u>Normal:</u> Sometimes experiences in life can change our personalities as we age.

10. <u>Loss of initiative:</u> Alzheimer's people can become very passive, sit in front of the TV watching test patterns, sleeping a lot, not wanting to participate in activities. <u>Normal:</u> Sometimes work or social obligations are a pain, but we usually follow through anyway.

LIVING IN AN EVIL FOG

There is very little accurate information about Alzheimer's in the public's mind. Most think it will not happen to them because they are well-educated, active mentally and physically, they eat right, exercise, and it doesn't run in the family. And, besides, they'd never forget their own children. Statistically, they are right, most people won't get it, but none of the above is any sort of guarantee that you can stave it off because, as of now, no one knows what causes it. Most who have it are like my husband was, he did everything right, there was nothing in his family (although in rare cases there is), or life style that might have caused it—nothing. Add to that, most caregivers are like I was; I really had no idea what I was dealing with. Almost any caregiver will tell you years after its onset that they wish they'd known at the beginning what they learned as the disease progressed.

I tried to imagine what my husband's mind must be like. I'd try to think of nothing, be a blank, unaware of what was going on around me, but I never really got close to what was happening to him internally. Yes, I saw the behavioral and physical changes, I was the object of his rages, I helped him with everything—eating, bathing, dressing—but until recently, I never really knew what it must have been like for him.

I think my son had a better idea than I did. I tend to be smart-alecky and flippant, say the wrong thing too many times, and one afternoon, as my husband was losing his ability to speak, I made a silly comment about him and my son said in an aside, "Mom, don't talk that way in front of him, he understands what you're saying." I knew immediately that he was right—I felt horrible. He was verbalizing less and less and I had fallen into treating him as a small child not yet

86

talking and unable to understand adult conversations. And he had no way to tell me about anything—if he was upset or offended—he was literally locked in a box of silence, but he still understood things. How could I have been so stupid and hurtful!

But, as time went on, I got better. I read more and more writings by people with early on-set Alzheimer's that gave me an insight into their feelings and were incredibly valuable in shaping my attitude and relationship with my husband as we traveled this difficult road together. I am so grateful—and, thanks to them, I did learn.

David Howe, 58, suffers from Alzheimer's. He and his wife, Elizabeth (Betsy), live in Lincoln, Nebraska. With her assistance, he has written what it feels like to live with this dreadful disease.

". . . . It feels like living in an evil fog. A fog is something all can understand. 'I' am inside. I can see out. I 'know' who I am and what I should be able to do. I 'know' what I want to say. But the fog envelops me. It holds me in its evil grasp. It keeps me from doing all I know I could before.

The fog sucks me in deeper and deeper, day by day, farther and farther from what should be my life. It's hard to watch myself leaving. It's hard for my wife and family to watch me leaving. I know that. I see that.

. . . . The right words more often won't come out of the fog. The fog grabs my ideas as they form and pulls them back into its evil clutches. By then the conversation has moved on without me.

The fog slows time for me and speeds up the outside world. Everything seems to move faster. I seem to keep moving slower. I daily trudge through a fog as thick as molasses. It sometimes gets exhausting and I must take a break with 'no brain' things, like reading or watching TV, but every now and then even reading or watching TV is exhausting.

. . . . 'What is' is 'what is.' I cannot change it. No one can change it. My wife helps me to continue to be 'me'. She helped me put together this article to share with you.

I hope that as the fog grows denser and pulls me farther and farther away, my friends and family will remember 'me'. I hope they will continue to talk to 'me' even when they can no longer see the 'me' clutched deep within the fog."

If you are moving through the minefields of Alzheimer's, unable or unwilling to understand why your loved one can't do what he did yesterday; can't remember that you answered that same question umpteen times already; can't find the kitchen; leaves doors open and water running; talks to 'someone' in the mirror; won't let you out of his sight; puts his shoes on the wrong foot; gets angry for no apparent reason; is unbearably slow; accuses you of stealing, being unfaithful—and on and on—then think of what it must be like to live inside that evil fog; unable to clearly communicate; getting lost in your own home; terrified of being left alone—almost any bizarre behavior is justified.

Understand that you cannot change your loved one's actions, all you can do is accept 'what is' and learn to adjust your responses. No one can tell you it's ever easy—no way! Read some books, join a support group, go on-line to research and communicate with others on Alzheimer's message boards who are going through the same stresses—you will learn and understand so much to make things a little easier—to know that **you are not alone**; keep a journal; seek help from Alzheimer's organizations and government programs. Nobody did anything wrong to bring this on, especially your loved one. Increase your compassion, try to be more patient with your loved one and yourself, be kind to both of you, and bless the Howe's and all those who must trudge through this evil fog.

(David Howe died February 4, 2010. He died as he lived. When asked how he was doing, Dave would reply, "I'm fine.")

MOM & DAD

Most of us really want to Honor our Father and our Mother. We want to take care of them; we love them and appreciate all the sacrifices they made to bring us to adulthood. *So why are they driving us crazy!* If your parents are cooperative and show gratitude for all that you do for them, drop on your knees right now and thank your lucky stars. Everyone else, read on.

No one likes to think about getting so elderly that we lose our independence, become a 'burden' to our children; and we adult children don't like to see our parents getting older, to see their fragility and becoming needy. Too often it happens when we are going full speed ahead with our own families, building a career, participating fully in our own lives. Or, when we finally have our children launched, we can retire, maybe travel; or beginning to display signs of our own aging and deteriorating health. It seems when we are the least ready, we have to begin a whole new passage in our own lives—just when we wanted to kick back and smell the roses.

Most elderly do not ask for help until there is a crisis and many adult children do not see the signs that something may be terribly wrong, especially if they live far away and visit infrequently. Too often changes are thought to be the result of aging, a common illness, or maybe just being tired and contrary—and sometimes it is. Nonetheless, the following should be given serious attention.

Someone is unsteady when standing, falls, has difficulty walking; lack of grooming, poor personal hygiene and wearing soiled clothing for days; changes in eating and cooking habits, spoiled food left around, loss of appetite, lack of food in the house or too much food that is not being eaten; the *biggie*—failing driving skills, dents and dings on the car, accidents or near misses; no interest in activities formerly enjoyed; reluctant to socialize; not concentrating, using poor judgment, memory loss, confusion and forgetfulness; another *biggie* is not taking medications properly, not taking them when scheduled or even double or triple dosing; lack of energy, always tired; sudden mood changes without reason, irritability; mail piled up, bills past due, checkbook a mess and money going out to whomever asks for it at the door, by phone, mail or TV; dirty house, unsafe conditions, normal general maintenance neglected.

You may have seen some of these things and wondered, maybe you saw something else or dismissed it all, but chances are you are feeling some concerns and don't quite know what to do. There is no 'one size fits all' response. This article is written for a 'typical' family—Mom, Dad, some adult kids and a dog. Since each family is unique with their own problems, personalities and life-long baggage, you will have to adapt it to your own. Maybe you were abused as a child and your feelings are hardly the same as someone raised as a perfect princess Daddy's girl or an adored little prince that the sun rises and sets in each day. So examining your own history and resultant feelings about caring for your parent, accepting how you truly feel and acting on that will clear things up a lot. Write a pro/con list if that will help. Is there resentment, guilt, duty or love and compassion; are you selfish, self-involved or outgoing and generous? Who was Dad's favorite and who did Mom never really like? All these things matter in how you will care for—or neglect—your parents and only you know how it is, only you can be honest.

Caring for an Alzheimer's spouse has its own problems, but caring for an elderly parent or loved one in a family setting, dealing with siblings and other relatives can be daunting, even in a close knit loving family with enough people ready to step up. Are you going to volunteer to be the caregiver? Consider whom you might be able to count on for help? You'll need it! Is brother a sweetheart or does he only stop by to see Mom when he wants money? Is there a sister-in-law from Hell? Who has small children, who lives nearby or far away? Can your parents move into someone's house, or can someone move into your parents' house? Who is likely to be their usual troublemaking self? Who can quit work to be an in-home caregiver? (Quitting work is often the wrong decision; it has to be carefully thought out, especially financially.)

All of these situations are generalities, you will have other issues but a family meeting is in order. Don't be surprised if some think there is nothing wrong—Mom and Dad are just getting old—some won't attend. Denial is a strong emotion when it comes to admitting your always powerful in charge parent is now in serious trouble. Too often, all the caregiving falls on the shoulders of one—usually a daughter. But it can be, and should be, a joint effort. Think about who can do what, talk about finances, divide up all that needs to be done, sharing is better than piling it all on just one. It's something for everyone to think about and express how they might contribute. Without support from others, after a time, the lone caregiver will suffer serious physical, emotional and mental stress; it's the nature of the disease. Alzheimer's is well known for taking down other family members along with the one who has it. While it often brings families together, it is not uncommon for it to destroy the family unit. Don't let that happen when it's the time that you will need each other the most.

If they haven't already been done, there are important things that must be taken care of. Because each state is different, you will need to consult an elder law attorney in your parent's state for Power of Attorney for finances and Durable Power of Attorney for Health Care to make medical decisions. Money has to be tied up so that it doesn't get spent foolishly by Mom or Dad. Any number of people thought there was plenty of money only to discover it was all gone—simply disappeared—when care was needed and there was no way to pay for it. Insurance has to be looked at, are premiums being paid, are Wills up to date; check out Social Security and any Veterans' benefits. A Living Will to explain the patient's wishes about possible end-of-life medical treatments can save surviving loved ones much anguish and guilt. Guardianship might be a possibility.

Begin to set the ground work for this, see that you are all on the same page; and, depending on the situation, you may or may not be able to do it without getting your parents involved. Now you have to speak to them—for most adult children it is a Herculean challenge that they want to avoid.

TALKING TO MOM & DAD

You've been watching Mom or Dad over time and think that one or both may have Alzheimer's. You fear that they can be in danger—driving, cooking, wandering—everything. They lack the ability and the will to make the necessary changes for their own well being. You need to talk to them about certain things—and it can be difficult. Parents often have a hard time listening to children. It's not easy to admit they need help and give up independence. Most say they are fine, always took care of themselves and always will. Hopefully you've talked to other family members about this and you're all on the same page. But someone has to take charge before there is a crisis—and there will be one. The relationship turns upside down, the parent becomes the child and the adult child assumes the parental role, you become your parent's protector. Many children have always been take-charge pushy, others have never been combative, always looking for a way to please. If you're the latter, taking control may seem impossible, but you can do it. Along with other family members, you might involve a minister, accountant, attorney or doctor in any talks. But don't gang up on them! Depending on what stage your parents are in, you cannot make definitive statements and think that you will be understood and agreed with immediately. You know they have cognitive problems, so work—gently and patiently—with that knowledge—it's sad and really hard for them—and for you, too. It is no longer safe for them to be left alone to do whatever they want, and remember that your needs are as important as theirs. Don't expect a normal response, although sometimes, if you're lucky, you may get a sigh of relief and gratitude.

Children do things they think parents never suspect, but in the adult world many parents have secrets and accepting help

94

from children can stress a parent's dignity when their financial, medical, family and social histories are bared. You have to be nonjudgmental when delving into their private lives. Maybe Mom doesn't want you to know she's been slipping money every month to your ne'er-do-well brother and losing $20 a week at Bingo. It happens.

Perhaps Dad's bills are not getting paid and you want to take over his finances, but he feels this is starting down a slippery slope to losing his autonomy. Stay positive; don't harp on his being unable to do things anymore. Tell him he should still be in charge, remain independent, and conserve his assets so that he won't have to ask for help later on. We all count on others for support, we can't always do everything alone, and you want to be part of his support, doing a little of his bookkeeping. Mention the idea of a Power of Attorney for finances. Ask whom he thinks might be good to represent him. Get a list of his assets, including bank account numbers, brokerage companies, safety deposit boxes, etc. Suggest someone's name be added to his checking account so that money can be used to pay emergency bills, if necessary, for rent, utilities, medical, and make a list of how his money will be used. Assure him his money will not be spent foolishly; promise to give him his bank statement every month for his approval. Get information about his accountant, attorney, insurance.

Some of you are rolling your eyes, thinking, 'Yeah, right! Not with my Dad.' You know your parents and what may or may not work. Such conversations do not always go well and it is better to drop hints and ideas from time to time rather than leap in with both feet. It can be a lot to deal with, so short little discussions are often best before things become combative, planting the seeds, suggesting you can talk about it more later on. Set specific dates when he can offer his input, get his opinion—hopefully the concept will begin to stick in his mind—and assure him that he still has control, making the decisions. Likely he knows he needs help, but denial may still be present.

Most people cannot or will not talk about some things. We are all going to die, and writing your Will does not hasten your time—I promise! When someone dies without a Will it is very hard on survivors, often creating situations that destroy lifelong relationships. You don't have to know—probably shouldn't know—details of what's in your parents' Wills, but explain how better it will be if they make a Will so that they have the final say on what is done with their assets and don't leave it for others to guess, argue about and decide the wrong way.

Regarding health care, most people think they'll call Mom's doctor, identify one's self as her child and get all her medical details. Well, maybe not. There is a Federal regulation, HIPAA, requiring that doctors and other care providers protect the privacy of patients. So Mom will have to sign a form stating who can talk with her doctor. Most hospitals and doctors have HIPAA forms, it's very easy, just ask.

For their own peace of mind, Mom and Dad should each have a Living Will, which has nothing to do with a conventional Will or a Living Trust that designates the distribution of property at time of death. Instead, a Living Will gives them the right to decide the type of health care they may, or may not want if they become incapacitated. They don't need medical knowledge for this. But it helps them to become familiar with medical care commonly given to patients seriously ill. Do they want life-prolonging treatments like drugs, feeding tubes, respirator, surgery, endless testing and everything else—or not? There are two givens: (1) No one knows what their future health condition may be, not every eventuality is possible to cover; and (2) no one knows what medical advances may occur. But a Living Will will keep them in charge as much as possible, and save their adult children a ton of anguish and grief.

If they are unable to make health care decisions, someone has to do it for them, and that requires a Durable Power of Attorney for Health Care. They appoint someone they trust to act as their surrogate or health care proxy to make necessary decisions for them and see that doctors and other health care personnel follow their expressed wishes. Otherwise, doctors are left on their own to decide by guess and by golly. With such documents, based on one's own expressed instructions, their personal agent will consider all options and make the best medical decisions for them deemed available at the time.

All these financial and health care things must be adapted to your own family, spouse or parent, and since each state is different, (documents can have other names), consult an Elder Law Attorney where the patient lives, hopefully, before dementia gets too severe. If you don't, these decisions might wind up in the hands of estranged family members, doctors, courts and judges who may not know what Mom and Dad preferred—and cost an awful lot of money.

SOPHIE

We have almost always had dogs. When the children were little, we also had rabbits, chickens, ducks, horses, turtles, fish, rats, canaries, guinea pigs, an occasional iguana, stray cat—whatever—and the backyard cemetery where many were buried. It wasn't a rural setting, just a house in the suburbs, a nearby stable and one or two animals at a time indoors or out. It taught responsibility, the reality of death, and the certainty that life goes on.

For a few years after my husband developed Alzheimer's we had no dogs and it was all much easier, I had enough to do. But the day came when I saw how empty his life was, how little he could still do and I decided we needed a dog. It would give him a focus, something to care for, to talk to without the stress of trying to follow a human conversation. So we went to the puppy orphanage where there were a couple dozen or more dogs assembled in the parking lot.

In the middle of them all was a big brown galoot standing head and haunches above the rest. "That one," I pointed. We walked 'that one' around a bit then took her to our car where she climbed right in, taking up all of the back seat. We had papers to sign, promising never to hit her with a rolled up newspaper, to bring her back if we didn't want her, never give her to anyone else, and on and on. It might be easier to adopt a child, but now she was ours and we all went home.

Her name was *Sophie,* a yellow-lab-German-shepherd mix, less than two years old. She quickly made herself at home, whoever had her before did a good job. She easily learned to communicate with us, to understand where her food bowl was, how to get out the back door and explore the house and yard. *Sophie* didn't seem like much of a name, so for a while I tried others, but people seemed to like *Sophie*, she responded to it, and as time went on, *Sophie* it remained. She had her own bed in our room, next to my husband's side—and it was all good.

She was great for him. He cleaned the yard after she decorated it, he gave her her breakfast—until the day I caught him putting prunes in her dish—and she'd bring him home if they went for a walk. One day we were all going for a stroll. In front of the house, my husband had her on a leash while I went inside for a sun hat. "Stay here," I told them, "don't go away." Moments later when I came back out, they were gone! I got in the car and began looking, asking everyone I saw if they'd seen a man and a big brown dog—I drove further and further, making bigger and bigger circles for a half-hour until I knew I had to call the police. I could not find them! But when I got home, there they were waiting at the back door, all sweaty and out of breath. I hugged and hugged them. "Where have you been?" I asked. "I don't know," my husband said—and *Sophie* wasn't talking. In the kitchen, they both gulped the water I gave them, I was so relieved.

Often we'd pile into my old car and I'd drive along the coast to watch the waves and stop at the wild duck pond where *Sophie,* with a bemused expression, would watch them all waddle around from the back window. Next would be a trip to the local hamburger take-out. *Sophie* understood when I drove up to order; she liked it because whoever was at the window would always say 'hi' to her when she'd poke her head out. Then we'd go to a little park and sit under a tree, the three of us sharing the food.

When I had to place my husband, I'd take her to the facility, but she didn't like it much. She was always well behaved, but I think there were too many nattering voices and hands reaching out to touch her, too many smells and metal walkers by her head. The patients all loved her, but by then my husband had declined and really didn't pay attention to her. The director always wanted me to bring her back, but I stopped.

When my husband finally left us, peacefully, *Sophie* was there with me, I was never alone. She was my comfort and my joy, a living, understanding, responsive presence in my home, in my car. Someone familiar I could talk to, to share memories and a deep love.

Sophie and I continued to grow old together. In doggie years we weren't that far apart. We both lost hearing, had trouble seeing, our legs were giving out, we both slept more. She went to the vet, I went to the doc, she had her pills, I had mine, and I believe she was getting doggie Alzheimer's—yes, there is such a thing! She could no longer get in the car without a man's lifting her in, she stopped eating, she was having 'accidents' in the house—and I know that bothered her. Finally, it was her time and I had to let her go to be with my husband.

This personal narrative aside, research indicates that pets can be a soothing influence with Alzheimer's patients both in the home and as therapy pets in hospitals, nursing homes and other care facilities. Studies at the University of Nebraska have shown that even a short-term visit by a therapy dog to a facility can ease agitation in those with Alzheimer's, that they are a useful adjunct to other calming activities, especially in the early evening when patients often become more upset and confused. Another study of people with Alzheimer's in a Veterans' Home showed that after a visit with a pet dog, they became more social, smiling, laughing, looking, touching and verbalizing. If you are a caregiver, a pet can be just another burden to take care of, but depending on your personal situation, it can also be a boon to you, your loved one and the family as a whole.

ALZHEIMER'S ASSOCIATION REPORT (1)

(Editor's note: Although these four segments are from a 2009 report and certain figures and specifics may have changed somewhat, they are still essentially applicable to the current situation and well worth the read.)

The Alzheimer's Association reports in 2009 that the healthcare costs for those 65 and older with Alzheimer's and other dementias are triple those for non-dementia people in the same age group. Medicare payments alone are almost three times higher and Medicaid payments alone are more than nine times higher for those with dementia than for those without dementia.

The country is facing unprecedented medical financial challenges with a rapidly aging baby boomer population. Alzheimer's already has an outrageous impact on Medicare and Medicaid, dwarfing everything else. The Association presents these numbers for the year 2004 to illustrate the disparity between costs of caring for those with dementias and those without dementias:

Average per person Payments	WITHOUT Alzheimer's or Other Dementias	WITH Alzheimer's or Other Dementias
Total payments*	$10,603	$33,007
Medicare	5,272	15,145
Medicaid	718	6,605
Private insurance	1,466	1,847
Other sources	211	519
HMO	704	410
Out-of-pocket	1,916	2,464
Uncompensated care	201	261

*Payments by source do not equal total payments due to population averaging.

People with Alzheimer's are high consumers of hospital, nursing home and other health and long-term care services which mean higher costs of Government programs and for millions of families. As families grapple with finances and states face budget shortfalls, Alzheimer's threatens to overwhelm both. Most people with Alzheimer's also have one or more other serious conditions such as diabetes or coronary heart disease. Alzheimer's can complicate the medical management of these problems and drive costs even higher.

In 2006, Medicare beneficiaries with diabetes plus Alzheimer's or other dementias had 64 percent more hospital stays than those with diabetes alone. An average Medicare payment for them was $20,655 while a payment for those with diabetes alone was only $12,979.

Those with coronary heart disease and Alzheimer's or other dementias had 42 percent more hospital stays than those with coronary heart disease alone. An average Medicare payment for them was $20,780 while a payment for those with coronary heart disease alone was only $14,640.

Families provide about 70 percent of caregiving for those with Alzheimer's and the on-going draining of finances ripples throughout the family and can be severe. In 2008, nearly 10 million Alzheimer's caregivers in American homes provided 8.5 billion hours of unpaid care valued at $94 billion. In addition to their unpaid caregiving, families have high out-of-pocket health and long-term care expenses.

Out-of-pocket costs not covered by Medicare, Medicaid or other sources of insurance are 28 percent higher for Medicare beneficiaries with Alzheimer's than those without. Individuals with Alzheimer's and other dementias living in nursing homes or assisted living facilities incurred the highest out-of-pocket costs, an average of $16,689 a year!

Today, there are 5.3 million Americans living with the disease and every 70 seconds someone in America develops it. *(Editor's note: Some patients never see a doctor for Alzheimer's and will not be counted in statistics, so there could be more.)* By mid-century someone will develop Alzheimer's every 33 seconds. By 2010, there will be nearly a half-million new cases each year; and by 2050, there will be nearly a million new cases each year.

Alzheimer's is the sixth leading cause of death in the country, the fifth leading cause of death among those 65 and older. From 2000 to 2006, while deaths from other major diseases dropped: heart disease down 11.5 percent; breast cancer down 6 percent; prostate cancer down 14.3 percent; stroke down 18.1 percent, deaths from Alzheimer's rose 47.1 percent.

(Editor's note: The evident rise in Alzheimer's deaths is somewhat due to changes in the Cause of Death on current Death Certificates. Embarrassment and stigma have kept people from admitting to Alzheimer's disease and Cause of Death was often listed as pneumonia, heart failure, or 'after a long illness.' More and more people are coming to understand that it is important to list 'Alzheimer's disease' as the true Cause of Death to garner accurate statistics, apply for and receive additional research funding, and teach the public that it is terminal.)

According to Harry Johns, Alzheimer's Association CEO, "Currently, there are no treatments that can prevent, delay or reverse Alzheimer's disease . . . . an aggressive plan is needed now to address the threat of this disease. There are too many lives, too little time and too much at stake for anything less."

ALZHEIMER'S ASSOCIATION REPORT (2)

Previously in (1), the extreme costs of Alzheimer's for Medicare, Medicaid and individual families, compared to other major diseases, was presented along with statistics on the projected massive increase in cases as the boomers age. The costs for Alzheimer's alone could easily bankrupt many medical programs and personal families. To date, there are no treatments that can prevent, delay or reverse the disease.

State budgets will suffer as well and in order to plan for this rapidly growing population, states must have reliable information about the characteristics and needs of their residents coping with Alzheimer's and other dementias. The Behavioral Risk Factors Surveillance System (BRFSS), in conjunction with the Centers for Disease Control and Prevention, is an existing survey to obtain this important information.

Caregivers in the states of Washington and North Carolina were allowed to say for themselves what their challenges are. In Washington, 48 percent of caregivers for individuals with memory loss or cognitive impairment revealed that <u>stress</u> was the greatest difficulty they faced. *(Editor's note: Stress is a major cause of illness in caregivers and the negative effects can last long after caregiving days are over.)* This year, an approved set of family caregiving questions is available for all states to add to their BRFSS survey and another set of questions on cognitive impairment is being developed for 2010.

The report also highlights the emerging role of mild cognitive impairment (MCI). Those with MCI have problems with memory, language or other essential cognitive functions that are severe enough to be noticed by the individual and others, but not severe enough to interfere with daily life. Although those with MCI have a higher risk of graduating to Alzheimer's, many never go on to develop the disease. Intervention with any disease-modifying treatment should occur as early as possible, ideally, even before symptoms occur and research on individuals with MCI may help to speed progress in finding ways to prevent or cure Alzheimer's and determine whether or not some treatments may work.

According to Ronald Petersen, M.D. Ph.D., the Alzheimer's Association's Medical Scientific Advisory Council Chair, "There is a rich, diverse variety of treatment possibilities for Alzheimer's that scientists are exploring, offering great hope that drugs that may slow or even reverse disease progression could be on the horizon."

It is common to confuse the definitions of 'dementia' and 'Alzheimer's.' The report defines it this way: <u>Dementia</u> is characterized by loss in memory and other cognitive abilities. <u>It is caused by various diseases and conditions</u> that result in damaged brain cells.

To be classified as dementia, the criteria must include at least one of the following: (1) Inability to generate coherent speech or understand spoken or written language. (2) Inability to recognize or identify objects, assuming intact sensory function. (3) Inability to execute motor activities, assuming intact motor abilities, sensory function and comprehension of the required task. (4) Inability to think abstractly, make sound judgments and plan and carry out complex tasks. The decline in cognitive abilities must be severe enough to interfere with daily life. *(Editor's note: Think of dementia as a symptom, like a fever. A fever can be caused by a ruptured appendix or an infected toe, but it is not an illness in and of itself. Dementia is a collection of symptoms that makes it difficult for individuals to deal with routine activities without some assistance.)*

The Association's report lists the most common types of dementia very briefly:

Alzheimer's disease is the most common type of dementia, accounting for 60 to 80 percent of cases. Individuals have difficulty remembering names and recent events. Early clinical symptoms can be apathy and depression. Later symptoms include impaired judgment, disorientation, confusion, behavior changes, and trouble speaking, swallowing and walking.

Vascular dementia (also known as multi-infarct or post-stroke dementia or vascular cognitive impairment) is considered the second most common type of dementia. Impairment is caused by decreased blood flow to parts of the brain, often due to a series of small strokes that block arteries. Symptoms often overlap with those of Alzheimer's, although memory may not be as seriously affected.

Mixed dementia is characterized by the presence of the hallmark abnormalities of Alzheimer's along with another type of dementia, most commonly vascular dementia, but also other types such as dementia with Lewy bodies.

Dementia with Lewy bodies is a pattern of decline that may be similar to Alzheimer's, including problems with memory, judgment and behavior changes. Alertness and severity of cognitive symptoms may fluctuate daily. Visual hallucinations, muscle rigidity and tremors are common.

Parkinson's disease individuals develop dementia in the later stages. The hallmark abnormality is Lewy bodies that form inside nerve cells in the brain.

<u>Frontotemporal dementia</u> involves damage to brain cells, especially in the front and side regions of the brain and cause changes in personality, behavior and difficulty with language. <u>Pick's disease</u> is one type of frontotemporal dementia.

<u>Creutzfeldt-Jakob disease</u> is a rapidly fatal disorder that impairs memory, coordination and causes behavior changes. <u>Variant Creutzfeldt-Jakob disease</u> is believed to be caused by consumption of products from cattle affected by mad cow disease.

<u>Normal pressure hydrocephalus</u> is caused by a buildup of fluid in the brain. Symptoms include difficulty walking, memory loss and inability to control urine. It can sometimes be corrected with surgical installation of a shunt in the brain to drain excess fluid.

(Editor's note: Dementia can also be caused by a blow to the head, alcohol and drug abuse, reaction to medications, depression, strokes, tumors, infections, allergies, diminished oxygen, nutritional deficiencies, any number of well-known diseases and more.)

ALZHEIMER'S ASSOCIATION REPORT (3)

Previously in (2), the most common types of dementia were briefly described, Alzheimer's disease being the most well known. As of now, no treatment is available to slow or stop the deterioration of brain cells in Alzheimer's. A handful of drugs have been approved by the Food and Drug Administration that may slow the worsening of symptoms for up to a year in about half of individuals who take them. As understanding the biology of the disease increases, researchers have identified strategies that may have the potential to change its course through therapies that are being clinically tested in volunteers.

Nonetheless, disease-modifying therapy studies consistently show active care of Alzheimer and other dementia patients can significantly improve quality of life through all stages for both the patient and the caregiver. These would include use of available treatment options, integration of managing any other coexisting treatments into a cohesive plan, and supportive services like counseling, adult day care, activity and support groups.

(Editor's note: There are some support groups for both the patient and the caregiver, together or alone, and I would add on-line support-groups. Caregivers often think their loved one is not ready for certain activities, feel that no one else can care the way they do, that their loved one will reject such activities—and sometimes they do. However, it's worth trying different options again from time to time as the illness progresses and the patient's attitudes change.)

One study found that people with less than 12 years of education had a 15 percent greater risk of developing dementia than those with 12 to 15 years of education and a 35 percent greater risk of developing dementia than people with more than 15 years of education. It may be that with more education, individuals have a 'cognitive reserve' that allows them to compensate for Alzheimer's and dementia symptoms. Achieving higher education may be due to socioeconomic effects. Where one lived, access to education, lower levels of occupational attainment and physical conditions in adulthood may also be associated with developing dementia.

Many scientists suggest that the health of the brain is closely linked to one's overall health. There are some indications that management of cardiovascular risks like high cholesterol, Type 2 diabetes, high blood pressure and being overweight may help avoid or delay cognitive decline. Regular exercise, low-fat diets rich in fruits and vegetables may support brain health, and even an active social life and mental stimulation may help.

(Editor's note: I'm in no position to challenge such findings by a coterie of scientists, however, my husband always had low cholesterol, low blood pressure and low blood sugar, he was naturally wiry, not overweight and had lots of exercise and mental stimulation in his work. We were both well educated, although I'm the one who, otherwise, has the most common markers for the disease. I don't think that's exceptional. It can't hurt to lead a healthy, active life style, to embrace education, but don't count on any of it to be a guaranteed safeguard. The Alzheimer's world is jam packed with people who were mentally and physically active and with the finest education—hardly a couch potato can be found.)

Women are more likely to have Alzheimer's and other dementias than men. Fourteen percent of all people aged 71 and older have dementia. Women have higher rates than men, 16 percent to 11 percent. Studies of the age-specific differences for men and women have shown no significant differences in gender. Essentially, women are more likely to have Alzheimer's and other dementias because they live longer. Gender is not a risk factor, but age is. Of those over age 71 with dementias, 70 percent are due to Alzheimer's; 17 percent are due to vascular dementia; and 13 percent due to other dementias.

The Association lists the help normally provided by family, universally unpaid, and as the disease progresses, the caregiving increases. It requires shopping for groceries, preparing meals, providing transportation; helping the person take medications correctly and follow treatment recommendations for the dementia and other medical conditions; managing finances and legal affairs; supervising the person to avoid unsafe activities such as wandering and getting lost; bathing, dressing, feeding and helping the person use the toilet or providing incontinence care; making arrangements for medical care and paid in-home assisted living or nursing home care; and managing behavioral symptoms.

Alzheimer's caregivers assist with all kinds of intimate personal care. They bathe the person 35 percent versus 25 percent of non-Alzheimer's caregivers; deal with bladder and bowel incontinence 32 percent versus 13 percent for non-Alzheimer's caregivers. These tasks are often made more difficult by the confusion, disorientation and agitation of the person with dementia who may be unable to cooperate and may even resist care. When someone with dementia moves to a care facility, the caregiver's help may change, but it is far from over. Many continue to take care of financial and legal affairs, make arrangements for medical care and to provide emotional support. They may also help with bathing, dressing, feeding and other personal care needs.

(Editor's note: As the sole 24/7 caregiver for my husband with Alzheimer's in our home for ten years, I can attest that it is a far more difficult task than anyone can imagine. From time

to time I had paid help in the house for a few hours a week, our adult children gave me respite on occasion, they were there for emergencies and stayed with him when I had to be someplace; briefly, he was in a care facility. Most caregivers do not get any help physically, financially or emotionally, it commonly falls on one person alone.)

ALZHEIMER'S ASSOCIATION REPORT (4)

Previously in (3), some of the disease-modifying therapies and support that the Association believes may make it easier for both the patient and the caregiver to better cope with Alzheimer's are mentioned. There were brief comments about brain health, gender and educational risk factors. The 24/7 stressful life of the Alzheimer's caregiver was described, and although caregiving for other medical conditions in the home can be every bit as daunting, the Alzheimer's patient is eventually unable to perform any personal task unassisted and the resulting confusion, disorientation and agitation make it doubly difficult and, indeed, often thwart the caregiver efforts at every turn.

Because Alzheimer's and other dementias often progress slowly, most caregivers spend many years in the role. At any one time, 32 percent of dementia family caregivers have been providing care for five or more years, while 39 percent have been providing care for one to four years. By contrast, 27 percent of caregivers to other elderly people without dementia provided care for five years or longer, and 32 percent have provided care for one to four years.

(Editor's note: It is not unheard of for Alzheimer's caregivers to be caregiving for seven to ten years, even 20. It depends on when the difficult behaviors begin to impact daily living, age at diagnosis, other medical factors, how fast the disease progresses, severity of symptoms, health of the caregiver, available help, whether or not the caregiver has small children or aging parents, and a host of other situations.)

Caring for a person with Alzheimer's poses special challenges beyond memory loss because the patient loses judgment, orientation, the ability to understand and communicate, and develops changes in personality and behavior. They require increasing levels of supervision and personal care causing many caregivers to experience high levels of stress and negative effects on their health, employment, income and financial security.

Most family caregivers are proud of the help they provide and some manage with little difficulty, but more than 40 percent of them rate the emotional stress as high or very high, and about one-third have symptoms of depression. In the year before a person's death, half the caregivers spent at least 46 hours a week assisting the person, 59 percent felt they were 'on duty' 24/7, and many felt that the end-of-life period was extremely stressful. Stress was so great, 72 percent said they experienced relief when the person died. One study found that caregiver stress, especially related to a loved one's behaviors associated with nursing home placement, was just as high after the person was placed as before.

(Editor's note: Notice that 46 hours a week is more than a full time job with no week-ends, holidays or vacations. Much of caregiving is what professional nurses do, but without such training, and no auxiliary staff to take care of all the other daily chores. They don't have a union to limit work hours, provide lunch times, coffee breaks and determine benefits and wages.)

Caregivers are more likely than non-caregivers to say their health is poor or only fair, and those caring for people with dementia are more likely than those caring for non-dementia older people to say that caregiving made their health worse. They are more likely to have high levels of stress hormones, reduced immune function, slow wound healing, new hypertension and new coronary heart disease.

Twenty-four percent of Alzheimer's spousal caregivers reported an emergency room visit or hospitalization for themselves. Spousal caregivers of those who were hospitalized for non-dementia conditions were less likely to die the following year than those caring for an Alzheimer's spouse.

One study of Alzheimer's caregivers found that 57 percent were employed full or part time. Of those, many went to work late, left early or took time off because of caregiving, reduced their work hours and turned down promotions. Eight percent quit entirely because of caregiving. Another study found those caring for Alzheimer's patients with behavioral symptoms were 31 percent more likely to quit work than those caring for non-Alzheimer's individuals, and 68 percent reduced their hours or quit.

Caregivers who turn down promotions, reduce hours and quit work lose job-related income and benefits, including employer contributions to their retirement savings. Those whose loved ones have Alzheimer's and other dementias use substantial amounts of paid care, some may be covered through certain public programs and private insurance, but family still must pay for much of it, averaging $216 a month, and long-distance caregivers have even higher expenditures.

(Editor's note: Caring for someone with dementia is expensive and physically daunting beyond understanding. Few have any real conception of what it involves, how it drains the well-being of anyone, no matter the circumstances, no matter how strong and careful one is or how sincere and hard one tries.)

Looking at the future, the Alzheimer's Association reports that research into the disease is evolving rapidly. We are learning a great deal about early symptoms and it is important not to ignore early warning features because the earlier we intervene, the better. Present 'intervention' might include education and knowledge about the course of the disease. With more research, recommendations may include information about lifestyle and even pharmacological interventions.

Memory impairment is a common complaint in the elderly and much has been learned about which types of memory complaints may be Alzheimer's or something else. Not all concerns about memory are problematic. Minor forgetfulness is common for most people and often increases with aging. It should not be interpreted to mean that Alzheimer's is inevitable. Ongoing neuroimaging techniques and biomarker studies will help identify the severity of disease in those with early signs of Alzheimer's.

(Editor's note: Alzheimer's disease is just one of many that have plagued the human race for thousands of years. Essentially I do not think that we 'cure' or eradicate most diseases, but we do a pretty good job of preventing them with vaccines and controlling their symptoms and severity with medications and other therapies. When society gets lax and overconfident, outbreaks of otherwise dormant conditions return, and in spite of all our flu shots, a new flu strain is developing even now. It'll take time, but we'll eventually get on top of Alzheimer's. Failure to do so is not an option.)

REPLACED AFFECTION
(PART 1 OF 2)

Supreme Court Justice Sandra Day O'Connor retired to be with and care for her husband, John, who has Alzheimer's. What surprised and upset much of the public was that her family went public with the news that John had fallen in love with another woman, an Alzheimer's patient residing in the same care facility. Ha! Countless Alzheimer's families were not at all surprised, it has happened over and over, again and again to any number of us. Welcome to the REALITY of Alzheimer's.

Most comments from the public were understanding, admitting that they didn't know this sort of thing happened. Some were hostile—*it's prurient, the media exploiting it, disgusting, sensationalism masquerading as educational, I'd never put up with that, I'd change nursing homes, not my husband! No how, no way!*

My story is typical. Shortly after I placed my husband, he and one of the lady residents got together. They were inseparable—they'd stroll hand in hand, she'd sit on his lap making out in the lounge, dine together, snuggle close—thigh to thigh. When I came to visit, she'd pull me away from him. At night she'd bang on his door wanting to get in. Staff told her he was married, but she'd yell, "No, he's mine!" My husband treated her with deference and great respect, introducing her to everyone as, "My wife, Betty Lee." Oddly, she didn't look like me any more than Abbot looked like Costello, but to him, she was his wife, Betty Lee. He was happy and I was happy for him.

Staff told me that they were used to this sort of behavior; they'd keep them apart if I wanted. I said to leave them alone. Others asked how I could stand it, told me what I should do. But, good grief, they were both demented! And I knew, as sure as I write these words, that he was not being unfaithful, through no fault of his own, he lived in another reality. I could rant and rage, *'how could you—after all I've done for you—this is how you treat me! Yada, yada!'* He'd just give me a bewildered look, wouldn't understand anything I said. I could tell her to keep her filthy hands off of him, scratch her eyes out, pull her hair—and get arrested for assault. No, it was OK, and if you understand, truly understand the REALITY of Alzheimer's, then you know it's OK, you understand.

Often enough patients recreate their own life in a facility doing what makes them comfortable. That's what my husband did. He wanted to be married to Betty Lee, and so he arranged it. I'd be foolish not to take that as an undying commitment of his love for me.

Try to find the movie, *"Away From Her."* The gender roles are reversed, but otherwise it's my story and O'Connor's as well. It's the caregiver spouse who is unceremoniously set adrift. Years of a 24/7 exhausting, frustrating, stressful life end abruptly. Depending on how things have gone, you can wake up suddenly alone one morning, bereft, in an empty house with the daunting prospect of establishing a new life—*alone*.

Adult children have their own grief and despair when the essence of a parent with Alzheimer's disappears. Difficult, uncomfortable feelings may arise when seeing their mother or father replaced by a stranger. That strong life-long bond to a parent who has always been there from the day of birth, and all that entails is gone. Never an easy loss—never at any age.

And it's not just wives and husbands re-establishing relationships. Often a person with Alzheimer's doesn't know their own children anymore and replaces them, bonding with a staff member who takes care of them. They create a new identity with the familiar face of someone they see all the time, remaking the family unit where they again find comfort, affection and nurturing.

My husband would give me the most loving smile, then turn the same adoring gaze to an aide who frequently helped him. Any number of caregivers can tell you that their loved one's affection has been transferred to someone else—if not another patient, then a caregiver in the home or a facility. Those with Alzheimer's constantly struggle with communication, memory loss and confusion; try to make sense of their lives and adjust any way they can. We have our reality and memories, but those with Alzheimer's have lost theirs, they are forced to deal with a new, frightening, strange world full of unknown people. In a normal world, someone's being unfaithful, forgetting their own children can be devastating, but the hard truth is that our loved ones with Alzheimer's no longer live in our world. They did not choose their destiny; they did not choose to leave. It is a kindness to allow them to make the best of whatever they have, wherever they find it, and whomever they find it with.

REPLACED AFFECTION
(PART 2 OF 2)

The personal aspects of replaced affection were discussed in (1), explaining how Alzheimer's patients try to restructure their lost lives with strangers to again enjoy the affection and comfort that the disease too often steals from them within their own family.

When a loved one has been placed in a care facility, it is not easy for the caregiver left alone trying to cope with the loss of someone's presence in the home, physically, emotionally and mentally. It is even more difficult when the loved one takes up with a stranger and develops a new physical and emotional bond, in effect, replacing the caregiving spouse.

It's all good and well to explain that it's the disease causing this behavior, not a conscious decision to abandon the spouse. True, one can realize that the Alzheimer spouse is finding comfort in a new relationship, feeling good, even happy, but it is not always easy for the caregiver's heart to accept. Understanding something intellectually does not mean that it is understood and accepted emotionally.

Such new attachments are not exclusive to a care facility; it can happen at home with a hired caregiver, it is not simply being unfaithful as we know it. The need to find new companions in the Alzheimer's world does not mean they've stopped loving us, those they've loved all their lives, they cannot control it, neither can we.

Why does it happen with some people and not with others? If and when it does happen, it depends on how the brain is working at any given point in the illness. Placed in a care facility, individuals are doing their best to find friends among strangers, others like themselves, to make sense of their lives. I've seen Alzheimer's patients in a care facility *talking* together with understanding, but it sounded all gibberish to me. Apparently they communicate well with each other, but not with someone like you and me, not with such ease.

When two people in a care facility form a bond, hold hands and carry on, it may not be exactly what we think of as *true love*. But it can certainly make each feel more comfortable; a hand to hold, a shoulder to lean on, hugs to give and receive can do a lot to make someone feel less lonely and abandoned in a new and unknown world. They must certainly suffer from separation anxiety. And, in time, as we all know, the patient's ability to recognize the spouse and other family members dwindles. The anxiety can be unbearable and a new friend, a new companion, a new relationship—whatever one may call it—can be a blessing to fill the void.

The adult caregiving child can feel the same loss when a parent is placed. Then they are further distraught when they see their parent/child lifetime bond so easily set aside. Both child and spouse caregiver can feel replaced. Years of suppressed grief surface, it's easy—it's natural—to be jealous. You did everything right and you still lost your loved one to a devilish disease. You can no longer continue all the physical and emotional work it takes to be a caregiver, and now you've lost your loved one all over again to a complete stranger who is getting all the attention and affection that is rightfully yours—that you've earned—you bet you're mad about it! And then someone has the audacity to tell you, 'Remember it's not personal, it's the disease!' Yeah, right, that makes it all better, all OK!

Most Alzheimer's patients need social connections just like the rest of us. The behavioral and emotional changes they are experiencing mean they respond and react to their new—and old—connections in different ways. Your loved one isn't rejecting you, it isn't that they don't care about you anymore; it's that they have lost their memories and feelings about someone they no longer accurately and truly remember. The familiar face of a family member will elicit a friendly smile, but there may be no memory of how that person, that face, now fits into one's life. Wife, sister, aunt, daughter, friend—it's just a familiar face—any one-to-one relationship memory is lost forever. It cannot be recalled, no matter how much prompting is tried. Of course, it makes it extremely difficult. One person has all the vivid memories, the other one does not and it's incredibly painful, few things are more so.

The sooner you internalize what is happening within your loved one's brain, the sooner you realize your loved one cannot help it—it's a matter of survival—then the sooner you will be able to accept and adapt. Countless family members have turned themselves inside out fighting and rejecting the reality of something they can neither change nor control. Learn to save yourself the anguish. *It really is the disease.*

There are community support groups and online resources available for family members. Counseling by a professional is often beneficial; someone who doesn't know either party personally will be more objective. Contact your local Alzheimer's Association to find help near you.

HOLIDAYS

Not everyone has an endearing Norman Rockwell childhood, but if we allow cynicism to slip a bit, most want to be with family, watching Mom set the Thanksgiving turkey on a holiday table. Everyone is gathered from far and near, happy, healthy, laughing—what a great day, and I was one of those lucky ones—every year—until I was a young mother myself and my Father died. I couldn't imagine a holiday without him, it wasn't possible. But the years passed and many happy holidays have since been enjoyed—10, 20, 50 years! Faces change, age, leave and younger ones come anew to the table, life just goes on, and all our anguish, all our tears and grief will never change that.

As my husband's Alzheimer's progressed, such events became more difficult, including birthdays, bar-be-cues on the Fourth, Mother's Day. I remember telling our children when our wedding anniversary came around that there would be no fuss. It didn't seem reasonable if one of us was completely unaware that the celebration was really meant for both of us. Yes, I cared, yes, it mattered, but I'd felt like a 'married widow' for some time, life was just topsy-turvy and after so many years, I had learned to live with things as they were.

When your loved one has dementia you are often worried about what is going to happen in a group. Will he disrupt the festivities? Anything might go wrong—a frightening outburst, saying inappropriate things, forgetting a grandchild, eating with fingers, getting up to roam aimlessly about—the possibilities, the embarrassments are endless. Hopefully you will be with caring people he knows and you have spoken to discretely in advance; alerting them so they will not be surprised and questioning. When my husband was quite advanced, we took him to our son's wedding and hired an aide to be nearby—just in case. My son, his bride and I had decided that if there was a problem, people would just have to understand. If the ceremony was interrupted, it would be resolved, they'd still be married. Alzheimer's was a big part of all our lives; it was accorded special accommodations, but not hidden away.

Too often it is hard not to dwell on how much things have changed from sweeter times, but a focus on making holidays as enjoyable as possible will help everyone. If you are hosting the event, your loved one may be able to help in the preparation, doing tasks that fit remaining abilities—just remember that things may be unfinished or not done to your liking, but it will make him feel useful, you can always tweak it later or settle for less than perfection. Can veggies be cut, tables set, packages wrapped, something stirred or put away? Yes, you'll likely have to get an earlier start and work slower to give your loved one time and direction, but he'll feel so much better, especially if you just accept and praise whatever he does as appreciated.

Blinking lights and large decorations that were not there the day before can confuse someone with Alzheimer's. Avoid lighted candles and artificial food, which is easy to mistake for something edible. Keep things simple, familiar and pathways clear. Let him help, keep him aware of changes and what's going on—even if he forgets—no surprises.

Television, lots of conversation and kitchen noise can stimulate and stress your loved one. Calm and quiet are best, try to keep your daily routine in place as much as possible. Prepare another room where your loved one can be alone and have a place to rest when things get too much.

If your loved one is in a care facility, plan to celebrate the holidays there. Most places have special meals and often accommodate small family gatherings. While you may want to bring him home, the facility usually becomes familiar to someone with Alzheimer's and a change of location can cause anxiety. Find out what activities are planned at the facility, ask how you can participate. Within months of placing my husband, he didn't even recognize our house when I brought him home.

During the holiday season don't descend to his room *en masse*. Plan for two or three people to visit on different days, even if he doesn't remember who they are or what day it is, they are likely to be welcomed anyway. Alzheimer's patients often have agitation around sundown. So schedule visits for his best time of day, maybe have breakfast or lunch rather than dinner.

Don't feel that you have to do everything that you or your mother always did. Pick and choose what means the most to you—simple and easy to do. So maybe you don't bake that special batch of Christmas cookies, it'll be OK. Simplify, ask others to help, to bring different dishes, use disposable plates and utensils. Take advantage of anyone who has offered to help—to shop, to tidy up, to stay with your loved one while you shop or get your hair done. Given enough notice, most people are glad to help. Maybe don't send out all those handwritten Christmas cards, with envelopes to address, stamps to add. An e-mail greeting may be just fine—it's the 21st century.

You know best what your loved one can tolerate and do. Don't be pushed by others into doing more than what's comfortable. Protect your loved one and yourself from too much stress, set boundaries, stick to them and enjoy!

THE OMBUDSMAN

Such a funny word—*ombudsman*, although it's easy enough to pronounce—only three parts *om-buds-man*. It's Swedish and literally means 'representative.' There is evidence that prototypes of ombudsmen were also functioning in the ancient world, but in modern times, in 1809 the Swedish legislature created a parliamentary agent of justice to serve as an intermediary between citizens and various government bureaucracies. The concept has since spread to a number of countries in the 20th century. Essentially, the ombudsman's job is to receive and investigate abuse complaints and to find ways to achieve a positive resolution. The ombudsman is usually independent, impartial, universally accessible, and empowered only to report and recommend, although sometimes they may mediate. Their duties and goals can vary greatly from country to country.

In the United States, ombudsmen are often found in corporations, universities, government agencies, newspapers, non-profits, and any number of common entities. Begun in 1972, the Long-Term Care Ombudsman Program, by law, exists in all states under the authorization of the Older Americans Act. They are advocates for residents of nursing homes, board and care homes, assisted living facilities and similar adult care facilities. Each state has an Office of the State Long-Term Care Ombudsman headed by a full-time state ombudsman. Thousands of local ombudsman staff and volunteers work in hundreds of communities throughout the country assisting residents and their families, providing a voice for those unable to speak for themselves.

State offices are funded by federal, state and local sources. Unfortunately, some states and communities have had to cut funding, but many volunteers, in addition to remaining paid staff, continue to serve facility residents.

All licensed skilled nursing and residential care facilities for the elderly are required by law to prominently display the Ombudsman poster listing services and contact numbers. There is no waiting list or fee for services. Look for the poster in the care facility where your loved one resides. If it's not there, see that it gets posted.

Individual ombudsman office services can vary from community to community, but ombudsmen are trained advocates, educated in the needs, rights and issues of residents, and knowing the local and state regulations governing long-term care facilities. They are skilled in working confidentially with residents and their families to meet residents' needs and improve their quality of life. They are mandated by state and federal law to visit care facilities for the elderly at least once a month, and investigate any suspected abuse or neglect.

Residents of long-term care facilities sometimes feel ignored or intimidated if they have a concern that goes unresolved. Many times when a problem is brought to light by the ombudsman, it is quickly resolved by the facility operator. In more serious cases, a report by the ombudsman to state licensing agencies may result in fines and penalties if it is substantiated.

Ombudsmen are charged with helping residents live as they wish. However, that may not be in agreement with what the family or facility thinks is best. The ombudsman will work to mediate a resolution that honors the expressed wish of the resident as much as possible.

Complaints may range from something relatively minor about cold food to more serious ones of short staffing, inadequate medical care and even outright neglect or abuse. The ombudsman will respond to each concern to improve the lives of all residents and help insure that they receive the highest quality care with the utmost dignity.

The long-term care ombudsmen safeguard quality of life. They can provide the security of having a caring advocate available even when a family member is not present or residents are afraid of repercussions if they complain.

Families are often relieved to know that help is available when problems arise and that they themselves can also learn from the ombudsman how to become effective advocates for their loved ones. Living in a care facility can be a very difficult time for the patient and the family, often there is no other reasonable choice but the ombudsman can help with transitions, mediate, explain and comfortably settle a variety of things by empowering residents and families. They restore that precious sense of dignity we all cherish. It is important to know that we are being listened to, that we will be treated well, whatever our personal limitations.

Take advantage of learning about your local ombudsman program. If you have a concern, go to them early on before something gets too bad and you have a hassle with the facility. In a long-term care situation you need everyone to get along as much as possible. Sticky problems that may be worrying you might well be resolved much easier than you thought.

CAREGIVING DEMENTIA

It was a perfectly ordinary day, I felt fine—and then something came over me. My head was buzzing, my entire system seemed out of whack, I had to sit down. What was wrong? We'd had a normal morning, breakfast, I gave my husband his pills, took my own—!!! Oh, no, what did I do!!! Back at the kitchen counter, I reenacted my routine, and sure enough, I realized I had mixed up our pills.

I called our HMO's emergency number, explained what I'd done, how I felt, and was assured that I would be OK. I was told to eat some bread, be patient, the effects would wear off. As for my husband, a little blood pressure meds, a touch of hormones wouldn't hurt him either and he didn't complain about anything.

The above scenario, my friends, is what is known as Caregiver Dementia and why some caregivers think that Alzheimer's is contagious when they, themselves, start doing wacky stuff, become forgetful and misplace things. Of course, perfectly normal ordinary people do things like this all the time and laugh it off. They rarely think they are getting Alzheimer's, maybe aging, but not a disease. It's when we live every day, year after year, with someone who has Alzheimer's, when we are constantly bombarded with such bizarre behaviors that we, obviously, think we may be getting the same disease when we do a normal silly thing like mixing up pills; I had done such things well before Alzheimer's came into our lives—and I'll bet you have, too.

Caregiving dementia is not a medical condition that you'd find in a medical journal. The term took hold in a caregiver chat room about ten years ago and has since spread throughout the Alzheimer's community. Those of us who have diagnosed it in ourselves understand that it comes about from unending, unrecognized stress compounded by sleep deprivation and neglecting our own well being. If you are the sole at-home caregiver to a loved one with Alzheimer's, that's the way your life probably runs.

Unrelenting anxiety and activity on the over-stressed caregiver will often cause it and a lagging mental state is ultimately experienced. Giving a non-technical name to some of the strange things you may say, do and think will lessen your worries, and assure you that you are not losing your mind that, eventually, you will return to normalcy.

I can suggest things to say and do to, maybe, lessen your stress, but I know from personal experience it is not always possible to follow such well-meaning advice. Still, it is worth telling that if you can find help for respite—take it. Do not continue to believe that you are the only one who can properly do the caregiving for your loved one. You can tell people that you are having a bout of caregiver dementia, what that means, that you are stretched to the max, angry, fearful, ready to collapse and if you don't get help—some time-off relief—you will end up in the hospital—a very real probability that too often happens. This is a REAL condition.

As an Alzheimer's caregiver, if you are frequently tired, needing to pause more often to get your thoughts back on track, recall a fact or word, this is not automatically the beginning of Alzheimer's, it's likely caregiver dementia. You have a valid reason to behave in such a fashion. Your concentration may suffer; you may be easily distracted and feel spacey. Find a quiet 'corner' that is just for you to relax without interruption—let any chores go—even a half hour will do wonders. You will need more sleep, try to eat better, consider a nutritional supplement, vitamins, and talk to your doctor who should understand the stresses of Alzheimer's caregiving and possibly prescribe a mild tranquilizer. If you do not address these stresses, take care of yourself—even a little—you will likely worsen, forgetting appointments, putting things in the wrong place. You will come to believe that your actions are like those of your loved one and you are, indeed, getting Alzheimer's. You can become moody, grumpy, (and you have reason to), think you are losing your mind, getting physically sick and not even realizing it. You need a break for yourself as well as your loved one. Haven't you already heard: *If you get sick, who will care for your loved one?* Well, who will?

Caregiving dementia can be a bit amusing in the beginning, but as time goes on, it can become serious. Recognize that you are only human; you cannot do it all alone. Think of the professional caregiver with years of training and experience who works all day then goes home to dinner, family, distraction and a good night's sleep. No matter our promises and vows, no matter our desires and need to be with our loved one, we ordinary untrained people cannot do it 24/7 without some respite, some relief from it all without serious consequences—and again, I speak from personal experience. I was aging with my own medical problems and should have sought more help, placed my dear husband sooner, although it broke my heart when I finally had to do it, I should have taken better care of myself. I realize that not all caregivers have other options, but far too often, what keeps caregivers from getting more help is in their own head. Think about it, and then think about it again, you don't have to do it all alone. Ask for help, accept it when offered. Caregiving for someone with Alzheimer's becomes incredibly daunting without your even realizing it. Remember that your life is just as important as your loved one, and you have the right to enjoy things, to let stuff go, to put yourself first from time to time—it really is OK.

HOME ALONE WITH DEMENTIA
(PART 1 OF 3)

Over twenty years ago I sat outside on the back steps of my Mother's apartment building crying. I had been called by a neighbor concerned that Mom was roaming around alone in the dark night. Other than her always having been a little difficult, I had no idea what was wrong with my Mother, but more and more her behavior was getting to me so I'd left my husband inside her apartment with everyone else, trying to calm things down. Now entering her 80's Mom had been living alone for several years and took good care of herself. My sisters and I took her shopping, to the doctor, things like that. We glossed over her getting her medicines mixed up, occasional leaking gas from burners not fully turned off, trouble with her checkbook. She was dressing properly, cooking her own meals, eating well, bathing regularly, doing laundry, house cleaning, and friendly with her neighbors—things were OK. True, she'd begun to call more frequently; I thought she was reaching out, so we'd talk, I'd drive over, find a reason to go to a store, just be together. It would be a long time before it clicked in my head that her elderly mother had done some of the same things a generation ago, a continent away, and I often heard that whatever my aunts tried to do to make things better, it always fell apart. That night I knew I could never leave Mom home alone again; we brought her back to our house.

Years earlier, after Dad died, Mom went to live with my oldest sister, but it didn't work out. So she had come to live with me, the youngest, there was no way she could live with the middle sister. She was a good mother; we were never neglected, hungry or cold, never abused; the absolute mother tiger, always protecting us, always on our side, and more understanding than we gave her credit for at the time.

But, but, but—she was impossible to live with in our marital homes. Our house was small; one bathroom and three little bedrooms. I wanted to put our two children in the same room and give Mom her own room, but she <u>insisted</u> that she'd sleep on the couch, not wanting to put anyone out, and obviously, that put us all out. My husband came home from work, wanted to take off his shoes, crash on the couch with a beer and watch whatever exhausted men watch on TV in our front room, but Mom was anxious to see Lawrence Walk—or she'd stand in the doorway holding her blankets and pillow, wearing her hairnet, ready to go to sleep for the night—and where were we supposed to go! All day long it was, "Betty Lee, where are the children? Its cold, do they have sweaters? Aren't you going to do those dishes? You need new curtains." This and that, that and this. My husband kept coming home later and later, the kids got confused. She would not—or maybe, could not—adapt to our household.

When she cracked her shoulder blade, it had to be all bandaged up, her arm in a sling to keep it from moving. But she kept undoing everything, trying to use her arm, letting it hang loose. I wrapped it all back together over and over. Finally I called the doctor and said that she had to be in a hospital, I could not control her and I feared she could do herself serious harm. Just keep her quiet they told me and don't let her use the arm. I'M TRYING, I CAN'T CONTROL HER! So she was hospitalized.

And so it came to pass, as it so often does, that good intentions are not always doable. We had our first and only ever screaming argument. It was either my marriage, my family or letting her run things. We found a bright sunny apartment for her about a mile from my house. After much recrimination, Mom actually came to like her little nest, her independence and for several years all went well—until the neighbor's phone call the night that I cried.

My sisters and I normally took easy turns caring for Mom and her needs. But they had been out of town; I'd been responsible for her all alone. When they returned I told them that I had to opt out—for my well-being, for my little family. It wasn't good for anyone to be sitting in the dark crying from sadness and frustration with no end in sight. My sisters were aging with their own serious medical problems. Things would only get worse. We decided to place her in an excellent nearby care facility. We wrote a simple agreement between us about how we would handle her finances and pay for everything to avoid possible misunderstandings. Again she fought it, how could we abandon her! But soon she enjoyed being there as well. We took her to lunch or shopping and still saw her as much as ever. It seemed that one Mother could take care of three children, but three children could not manage to personally care for one Mother, try as they might.

Many caregivers are all alone, there's no help and not enough resources. Some people refuse to spend any money on caregiving; others may live a distance away or be indifferent to the needs of the caregiver and the patient. But the biggest hurdle is often the elderly person who is uncooperative. Hire someone to be in the house and they fire them. Explain that it is not safe for them to live alone, and they counter that they are just fine, always took care of themselves, always will. They don't want to leave their home (neither would I), they don't have money for a caregiver or a care facility; they say the neighbors look after them, etc. They are fighting to hold on to what they have of their personal lives, keep their independence—and who can blame them? But it drives everyone who feels responsible for them a little nutty—waiting for some sort of disaster to happen. How do you know when someone should not be left home alone, it's rarely easy to tell and even harder to do anything about it.

HOME ALONE WITH DEMENTIA
(PART 2 OF 3)

Having described the problems my family had with my elderly mother's dementia and the resultant trauma that happens, there is little to be done to avoid it. The best anyone can hope for is to recognize the events and handle them in the most reasonable way possible.

We are all living longer and longer—few would choose it to be otherwise. But as we age, dementia problems increase and leave many of us in the untenable position I was in with my Mother; and I know that millions of people are going through the same script in their family homes right now. Further, after Mother died, I took care of my dear husband with Alzheimer's for ten years until the time came, in spite of my best efforts, when the body simply said, 'no more' and I had to place him in a care facility. He could not be left alone—not even for a minute—not ever—I could no longer do it all. It broke my heart.

My eldest sister died at 90. We had a caretaker in her house for the last month or so—she became frail with old age. Until then, she was playing poker and winning, no dementia, thankfully. The middle sister, now 88, has definite dementia—like our Mother and Grandmother—not sure just why, again it's not Alzheimer's, although many of the same symptoms occur. Three direct generations of intelligent but difficult women, maybe more, developing dementia when they become elderly. From odd little events my sister has described, my layman's guess is that she has had some unrecognized mini-strokes over the years. Fortunately, she gave up driving on her own—had too many fender-benders—she was aware. Her son is arranging for someone to stay with her—she is resisting—doesn't want to give up her independence, and no one blames her—but she's getting worse.

If you find yourself in a family situation like mine and think that you should not leave your loved one alone, it's a good idea to pay attention to that feeling. But how do you know, what are the signs that give you a clue?

<u>First and Foremost</u>: It is very easy to think that your loved one is putting you on. I look back now and remember that my sisters and I often thought my Mother's behavior was more a call for attention than that she was really having problems with certain things. She had always been difficult and clinging, it naturally followed that we'd feel that way. Maybe part was for attention, but some of it was certainly dementia's setting in and we didn't see it, didn't understand. So it behooves you to try to sort it out. Chances are your loved one is <u>not</u> faking. You may be saying: *'Yeah, but you don't know MY loved one!'* I'm just saying: *'Think about it.'*

Those with dementia often seem perfectly normal, but many disabilities are hidden in their condition that can lead to dangerous situations when home alone. A home alone problem, adapt for spouse or parent, is likely in the making if any of the following is familiar.

♦ You've got that uncomfortable gut feeling!
♦ Loved one is acting fearful, you'll see it in the eyes.
♦ Upset when you've been gone even a short time, asking where you've been for so long.
♦ Hiding things, paranoia.
♦ Accusations of infidelity.
♦ Tools being used unsafely.
♦ Goes out looking for you, especially in extreme weather or in the car.
♦ Phoning everyone to find you.
♦ Takes medication when you're not there.

♦ Doesn't eat the food you've left.
♦ Water, gas, heat, appliances left on, doors left open and unlocked.
♦ Things have been moved out of place for no apparent reason.
♦ Loses a sense of time, doesn't know what to expect next, panics.
♦ Unable to sequence to plan an activity, gets frightened, frustrated.
♦ Cannot follow simple directions.
♦ Making a sandwich or a cup of coffee become confusing.
♦ Puts things in inappropriate places.
♦ Unable to find things in the house—like the bathroom.
♦ Unable to do everyday tasks always done before.
♦ Written signs and lists are too difficult when unable to read and comprehend.
♦ No insight into personal disabilities, refuses in-home assistance, will send help away.
♦ Loss of a sense of danger and risk.
♦ Trouble with the checkbook and making change.
♦ Cannot respond properly in an emergency.
♦ Wandering outside aimlessly, maybe looking for someone or someplace.
♦ Keeps asking to go home when already at home.
♦ Whatever else makes you uneasy!

People get sick; family takes care of them when they can. It just isn't always possible. Some caregivers need to work, there can be more than one person in the family who needs constant caregiving, small children in the house consume attention, caregivers often have their own medical problems, aging takes its toll. About 15% of Alzheimer's caregivers die before their contemporaries and too often before their loved one.

For help and guidance with home alone problems, go to your phone book or computer to contact Adult Protective Services; and the Alzheimer's Association that often has information about other dementias as well, but it may differ from office to office. In the County where your loved one lives, contact entities like geriatric care managers; senior centers; senior nutrition; health services; aging department or aging administration; mental health; care and aid for the aging; council on aging; elder abuse—whatever looks like a source of possible assistance. It will take time and false leads, but keep asking everyplace and everyone—with perseverance and luck you will get help.

HOME ALONE WITH DEMENTIA
(PART 3 OF 3)

About five years after my husband's diagnosis we were still doing OK—or so I thought. His accusations about my divorcing him and being with other men were ongoing, his hostile aggression toward me was increasing, he was having trouble doing things he'd always done before and he'd begun to talk about his dying—said that he had nothing left to live for. He worried about how I'd get along financially without him and he clung to me like my shadow.

I'd had a severe case of shingles, was hospitalized with a skull fracture from a bad fall, (until then, I'd always been sure-footed), and I had emergency surgery for a ruptured appendix. For someone healthy and strong, things were not going all that well for me but, recovering each time, I always felt fine and in charge. While I had some concerns that I'd have to make plans for his care if something really serious happened to me, we were still pretty much just plugging along, doing what we always did but in an increasingly restricted way. ***What Was I Thinking!***

I'd fallen so softly into the Alzheimer's caregiving trap that I hardly noticed how profoundly things had changed—which brings me to the last time I ever left my husband alone. I'd gone out to do some errands and when I returned home my husband was consumed with sheer terror. He had out my personal phone book, papers he'd written confusing notes on, he'd been trying to call everyone he could think of. He panicked, "I saw you at the border, I thought you were leaving." (We live just a couple hours from Mexico.) He was saying things that made no sense and I realized I could never leave him home alone again, it would be too heartlessly cruel, his fear that he'd be alone, abandoned was completely overpowering him.

But caregivers need to do things and cannot always take a loved one along. So I hired a man from the senior center to be my husband's companion on occasion. He resisted at first, but then enjoyed the visits. They went to the park, a museum, ate lunch, walked—had man talks and stuff. If not the senior center, caregivers might find someone from church, a neighbor, or reliable college student who would be available to help—and maybe adult day care.

Those living alone present a different problem. They often say neighbors look out for them, and neighbors might 'look in' but seldom have the time, experience, patience and understanding required for an on-going basis. It's hard when you are responsible for someone who is living alone to move them to a safer environment—especially if they live far away. Those who lived isolated lives may refuse to move closer to assistance, or maybe they can't. Lack of resources and fragility can be present but pride, stubbornness, fear, anger, independence, embarrassment and more keep some from asking for the relief they need. For possible assistance, look in the phone book or a computer for a geriatric care manager.

Maybe you want to move your loved one into an apartment near you, but if they can't cope alone in their familiar home, they won't be able to do it in a strange place. If you take them into your home, it may work out well; or the challenges could be endless. Do you work, have stairs? Who is more important—spouse, parent, children—you? Can you stay up half the night when they wander the house? There are endless errands, doctor appointments, phone calls, clean-ups. How many years can you do all that? Will your marriage falter; will you miss your children's school events, a social life?

Families often reject care facilities fearing placement will hasten progress of the disease. It rarely does although there may be a set-back adjustment to a new place; and there's worry that care will not be sufficient. Finding a good facility (they do exist), preparing for a smooth transition, being involved with staff and keeping a careful eye on your loved one may not be the worst option to someone's being home alone with dementia.

Take advantage of the knowledge and experience of millions who have lived, studied, treated and written about dementia. Many of the foundations below have brochures to help you better understand the illness. Be aware, too, that terminology continually changes so you might have to search around a bit to find exactly what you want. That's a good thing; it indicates that research is clearly making more definitive discoveries. Pick's disease now falls under FTD; stroke and multi-infarcts can be part of VaD; genetics may be involved; sometimes more than one malady appears in the same person. Things are not always clear cut. No wonder it's so difficult to get a definitive diagnosis!

Learn what you are dealing with!

Dementia: emedicinehealth.com/dementia_overview/article_em.htm

Frontotemporal dementia (FTD):

        ftd-picks.org/frontotemporal-dementias 1-866-507-7222

Pick's disease: nnpdf.org 1-877-287-3672

Lewy body dementia (LBD): lewybodydementia.org 1-800-539-9767

Alzheimer's disease (AD): alz.org 1-800-272-3900

Vascular dementia (VaD): medscape.com/viewarticle/452842_2

Mixed dementia:
  janssen-ortho.com/JOI/pdf_files/060686_07eCR_Leavebehind.pdf

---

A DECENT DIAGNOSIS

You have gone to a doctor because your loved one has been getting forgetful, making strange decisions, saying odd things; you know 'something' is wrong and yet, there's nothing you can put your finger on. It is often difficult to get a decent diagnosis for Alzheimer's, to understand what is happening, what *will* happen and what to do about any of it.

Alzheimer's may have crossed your mind; you pray it's not *that!* And you feel a sense of relief if you're told that it's depression, stress, aging. There may be a medical exam, asking a few memory questions, taking blood and urine samples, ordering a brain scan. Maybe you're told it's mild cognitive impairment, short-term memory loss or *'probable'* Alzheimer's—isn't it one way or the other!

Other than Alzheimer's, countless situations can cause dementia; accidents, a blow to the head, tumors, alcoholism, allergies, aging, anesthesia, vitamin deficiencies; and brain conditions like Creutzfeldt-Jakob disease, Huntington's disease, Parkinson's disease, Pick's disease, Wernicke-Korsakoff syndrome, Frontotemporal dementia, Lewy Body disease, vascular disease and more. While the causes may be different, common symptoms often overlap resulting in a misdiagnosis. It is not unusual to have a diagnosis of Alzheimer's and then two years later have it changed to something like Frontotemporal dementia—or the reverse. New tests keep coming on line that are making diagnosis more accurate, 85% to 90%, but it can still be very fluid.

Most doctors are compassionate, really do care, and patients and their families are entitled to a complete, dignified diagnosis. But too often after the visit, they leave feeling that things were left incomplete. *(First time at our doctor's office, I said that I didn't want to hear the word Alzheimer's—a personal defensive decision.)*

The Alzheimer's Association asked people with the disease what they and their families need and want from a diagnosis. Here are some of their comments. Your thoughts may differ—do what feels comfortable for you.

▶ Talk directly to me, the person with dementia; my family will also be affected, but I need to know first.

▶ Tell the truth. If you don't have the answers, be honest about what you do or do not know.

▶ Test early to help me cope and get information sooner about things like clinical trials.

▶ Take my concerns seriously, regardless of my age. Don't tell me 'you're just getting old.' Alzheimer's can affect those in their 40's or even younger; don't tell me 'you're too young.'

▶ Speak in a plain but sensitive way. Use non-medical terms that I can understand and be sensitive to how it may make me feel.

▶ Coordinate with all my care providers. I may be seeing other doctors. It is important that you share information and avoid my having to take unnecessary repeat tests.

▶ Explain the purpose of the different tests and what you hope to learn. Testing is physically and emotionally difficult. Tell me how long tests will take and allow me to take breaks, if possible, and to ask questions.

▶ Give me tools for living with this disease. Don't give me a diagnosis and then leave me alone to deal with it. I need to know what will happen, about medical treatments, and what help is available through the Alzheimer's Association, other organizations and resources in my area.

▶ Work with me on a plan for healthy living. Medications may help the Alzheimer's symptoms, but I need other recommendations to keep myself as healthy as possible through diet, exercise and social engagements.

▶ I am an individual and the way I experience this disease will be unique. I have been told that, 'When you see one person with Alzheimer's, you've seen ONE person with Alzheimer's.'

▶ Alzheimer's is a journey. Treatment doesn't end with writing a prescription. Be my advocate—not just for my Alzheimer's care, but for my quality of life.

Alzheimer's is a progressive brain disease and the physical, emotional and social implications of the diagnosis need to be considered throughout its course. Doctors have a world of people to care for but, inasmuch as possible, it is imperative that they develop a greater understanding of Alzheimer's and strive to keep a close relationship with the patient and caregivers. Too often families feel abandoned while trying to maintain a normal life. For now, there is no cure or prevention; and statistically, more and more people will be getting Alzheimer's and finding their way to a doctor's office.

Bookstores are overflowing with Alzheimer's books—read one—especially if written by a non-professional caregiver. And, if doctors have not had intimate personal experience with the disease or have not studied it in training, a book or two will give them valuable insight into it and a better understanding of what the patients and family go through. *Not all knowledge comes from lectures and labs.*

EDUCATING THE MEDICAL WORLD

In June 2001, the Alzheimer's Association conducted an on-line poll asking, "Do you think your physician is knowledgeable about Alzheimer's disease?" Over 62% of respondents said, "No." I was not surprised. In the decade I cared for my husband, I interacted with many doctors. A few were helpful, several understood the medical mechanics of the disease but had no idea what went on with the patients and caregivers outside of the office, some would have steered me wrong if I had listened to them, and others simply had no clue.

Many practitioners have never seen Alzheimer's and even if they have, they really don't understand what it is, how it permeates each and every crevice of the patient's life, including the lives of all family members. It's not a disease like cancer—which is bad enough—because in addition to the deep fear and sorrow there are mental and emotional flare-ups that destroy relationships, hurt feelings, violent rages and misunderstandings that create anger and divisions among people who have always been loving and close. Friends stop visiting, children and family turn away, divorce happens—it's not surprising that doctors can also be dismissive.

In addition to the physicians one sees for Alzheimer's, there's the dentist, eye doctor, podiatrist, proctologist, ear-nose-and-throat, heart specialist—on and on. My husband knew our long-time dentist well and the dentist was aware of his condition, but as time went on it became increasingly difficult for him to care for my husband's dental needs. There was fear, fidgeting, refusal or inability to understand even a simple 'open wide.' Poking and probing the body orifices of an Alzheimer's patient is bound to create impossible problems, especially if the examiner does not understand dementia. So it has been my mantra for years that **'*everyone entering any medical field should be required to take a course in how to work with dementia patients.*'** Sooner or later they are going to interact with someone who needs special attention—at least give them a 'heads up.'

My husband was going to have colon surgery and a counselor at UCLA told me that it would be best for me to stay with him 24/7 and that I should talk to the surgeon and anesthesiologist beforehand about my husband's dementia. I arranged a cot for me in his hospital room, but the pre-surgery talks did not go well. There was no interest in what I had to say. Clearly, I was a busybody getting in their way. My input ignored, the surgery went well; I waited in his room for him to fully wake up and the fun to begin.

He thought he was in a hotel, didn't know he'd had surgery, bewildered, he kept pulling and twisting the IV tubes. He tried to get out of bed to use the bathroom, didn't understand about the catheter. The nurse showed him the buzzer to call for a pain pill—he smiled 'yes,' but had no idea what to do. When the surgeon asked how he was doing, my husband pointed to his right shoulder, talking about some imaginary tumor—not the incision in his abdomen! The surgeon seemed not to notice his odd response. I explained to everyone about dementia, that you could not rely on his answers, that he could not use the buzzer, could not unwrap the food they eventually brought, could not follow directions, would pull out tubes, get out of bed, walk away—please talk to ME, listen to ME. Again I felt like an interfering biddy. Why didn't they acknowledge his inability to respond properly!

If you are a caregiver—or even just casually aware of someone with Alzheimer's, understand that *they cannot reason, cannot learn new things, forget how to do lifelong tasks—like brushing their teeth, using the toilet, bathing, dressing, eating, reading; they confuse language—will say 'yes' for 'no,' cannot physically respond to 'stand up' or 'sit down,' visual perception changes.*

145

They are not pretending or trying to annoy you. It is so hard because they behave normally much of the time. And those who see them occasionally, like doctors, really do not recognize that their behavior is not normal. As the disease progresses, you will have to be their advocate, reason for them, respond for them, maintain their memory for them, teach the world.

One out of three Americans knows of someone with Alzheimer's. How much do *you* know about it? You can help by educating yourself and the public, including those in the medical field who interact with Alzheimer's patients but often do not comprehend their behaviors and the resultant chaos that reigns in the home. You will often be ignored and rebuffed but at least a seed gets planted. Alzheimer's is not going to go away, not for a long, long time.

JUST ANOTHER SCAM

Maybe you've already heard about this—just another scam—but it happened very close to me. I live in California and rent rooms to college men from a nearby university. They come from all over America as well as foreign countries. David is from the mid-west and we were just chatting a few days ago when his cell phone rang, it was his grandmother. Hurriedly, she told him she was trying to get the money for him and hung up. She didn't answer when he called her back, so he phoned his parents who had no idea what was happening. I will try to tell the story as factually as I can because I was never certain exactly what was going on, but essentially, this is it.

His grandmother still drives and lives alone. For the most part she takes good care of herself, although sometimes she's a bit vague—but then she is 87—getting old, you know. They think she's OK, but maybe they should do something—just not sure what or when. And then they got this strange phone call from David.

When his parents called her house, she doesn't have a cell phone, she didn't answer, so they began to look for her and because she'd told David she was trying to get money for him, they went to her bank, and, yes, she'd been there. She wanted them to send $3,000 to Western Union in Canada because her grandson, David, was in jail and she had to get him out. She said David had told her he'd gone to a wedding, got drunk, was driving, had an accident and was in terrible trouble—and don't tell his parents! It would really make his dad mad. The bank told her they thought it was a scam and refused to do it, but she withdrew the money and said she'd do it herself.

His parents then went to Western Union. Yes, she'd been there, too. They also said it was a scam and refused to send it. She told them David's attorney said it had to be sent right away. Then she left and they didn't know where she'd gone.

She doesn't understand about cell phones. When she called David, he was standing in my kitchen. But she was unable to put that together, she thought she was talking to him in a Canadian jail cell.

Now David's parents didn't know where she'd gone, so they went back to her house, hoping she'd be there and she was. She was relieved that she'd finally sent the money and showed them the receipt from a different Western Union. They immediately called and were able to alert the Canadian office not to give anyone the money. I never found out what happened in Canada, maybe the scammers felt something had gone awry and didn't show up, or maybe they did and left empty-handed. Whether the Mounties were ever told, I don't know. I can't verify the details, but I was there when she called David and if she hadn't done that, it would have turned out quite different.

I have a grandson much like him and if someone called me and said it was him and he was in jail, I think I would have known his voice, but maybe not. It would be terribly frightening in any case, especially for an elderly lady. Scamming the money was bad enough, but to scare her that way is simply cruel. Anything could have happened to her. Fortunately, the family is now stepping in.

It's a warning to those who care for someone with dementia. Restrict access to money and credit cards. If it doesn't go to a scam like this, it can all go to a religious TV show, or a phony charity, someone at the door selling a new roof, whatever, someone will think of something. I know I've been scammed and so has nearly everyone I've ever asked about it. Fess up now, how 'bout you?

And if you have a computer, don't send any money to Nigeria, no matter what the story. Don't send money to some handsome/ beautiful person, (it's not their real photo, anyway), who is madly in love with you, but suddenly has an emergency, needs money that will be paid back and then, because you're so perfect for each other, you'll be married and live happily ever after.

Lists of elderly people get sold and passed around all the time, it's big business. All a scammer has to do is look at such a list of people over 60 or so, call all the women, and chances are that they will hit a grandmother. Everyone thinks it can't happen to them—until it does.

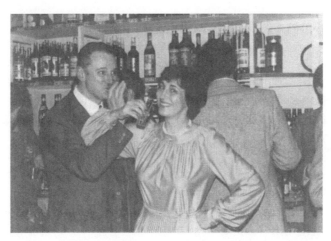

Pierre and the author in his *cave a vin*,
Southwest France.

PIERRE

Pierre died last night. Pierre lived his 84 years in a Bearn French village sheltered by the Pyrenees about an hour from the Spanish border as his *pere* had done, and his *pere* before him, and his *pere* before him for hundreds of years. He was the *proprietaire* of a small family wine business that had been handed down for generations and servicing the southwest region. Pierre was waiting outside his *cave a vin* for us, hatless on a cool breezy April day. *Americains* from *Californie! Bonjour, bonjour, bienvenue,* come inside where it's warm, sit down, sit down, *aperitif?*

And so I entered Pierre's world, his wine store that had obviously been the carriage house decades before with living quarters upstairs. Bottles and racks, labels and wine. Across a narrow street, in an ancient building, its original purpose long forgotten, was a little bottling plant, glass clinking as bottles rode around the conveyer, receiving their labels, gulping corks. It was so small compared to what I was used to, almost like a toy, but it did the job. Through an opening in the back was a chilly *cave* where boxes of wine were stored. It all had a certain warm charm that made me smile inside.

Pierre was a happy man, hale and hearty, tall and burly for a Frenchman. He, his family, melded with the village. Everyone knew him, admired him. He was active in all the village activities. But his English was non-existent, could not manage, 'hello,' and my fractured French just got me into trouble and afforded everyone a good laugh whenever I tried to speak.

In two years our lives would be forever entwined as his son married my daughter in the 11ᵗʰ century village church where a timeless string of men played a never-ending game of *pelote* on its exterior back wall.

Not long after that he lost his adored wife, and I don't think he was ever really happy again. Oh, he tried, but the sadness was always there in his eyes, and when my husband later died from Alzheimer's those eyes told me, without any needed words, that he understood—we understood each other. Every year I'd visit France and always return to the village and commune again with Pierre. In due time we shared two grandsons, little Franco-Americans we watched together with pride and joy as they grew into the finest of men.

And then, maybe five year ago, Alzheimer's evil cousin, Parkinson's, came upon him. Now there was more to share that neither of us wanted. Both diseases are distinct neurological degenerative disorders. One-third of Alzheimer's patients develop Parkinson's, and some Parkinson's patients develop signs of Alzheimer's. Scientists have considered for years if there might be a link between them and increasingly research studies seem to imply there is a possible connection. Eventually Pierre needed fulltime care; he was placed in a facility, and finally moved to palliative care and died in peace and comfort.

Parkinson's is incurable. It steals the motor functions of a person that causes a trembling or palsy to dominate the body. Difficulty with balance and walking appears resulting in more trips and falls, a serious consideration for someone's well being.

The diseases are dissimilar in that Parkinson's concentrates more on physical handicaps while Alzheimer's attacks mental abilities prior to deteriorating motor and physical skills. Although the ultimate causes may be different, symptoms of both diseases can be very much alike and possibly develop along the same lines.

I could see the results of the disease on Pierre, but mostly heard about it from others. The last time we sat across from each other at lunch he poured my wine, something he's done throughout his life. He was shaking so that I wanted to reach out and steady his hand. Would it spill, would something break? But I held back, he smiled, it was OK.

Rest easy, *mon ami.*

THE EMERGENCY ROOM (ER)

I was maybe eight when a playmate accidentally pushed me through a glass door, slitting my left wrist. Surprised and fascinated, I watched blood pump out of the artery, not understanding how serious it was, while a man put a tourniquet on my upper arm and called an ambulance. There was no pain or fear, but I was thoroughly impressed with the speeding ambulance and its siren. Just as well—I had no idea what was going to happen. On the operating table, I caught bits of conversation as my hand was bound down. *"Internal stitches—sewing inside—veins, artery, nerves—stick her palm—feel that? No, she has to feel—fingers moving?"* A nurse soothed my head, "I know it hurts, honey, just a few more minutes." If you were around that day, surely you heard my screams and it felt so good to scream. Finally, with three or four outside stitches, I left the ER—and still carry the scar.

Pretty routine ER care, but you can't count on its going that way when the patient has Alzheimer's and one never knows when an emergency may arise. It helps to be prepared. Make a list and start with the patient's primary physician and any specialists with their phone numbers and anyone who has legal permission to discuss medical problems. Include a summary of patient's dementia condition and any other health problems, allergies, all medications, vitamins and supplements, including dosages. Have copies of insurance, Medicare, Medicaid or HMO enrollment cards. Most of this can be typed on one page and kept in your wallet. Give the list to others who also provide care, including facilities like adult day care and anywhere your loved one may frequent without you.

You may also have things like a health care proxy, advance health care directive, living will, power of attorney and 'do not resuscitate' order, documents not easy to carry around, but at least know where they are in the house if someone has to go get them. If you and your loved one are both in the ER because of something like an auto accident, you may be unable to participate, so have your identification in your wallet with numbers of two or three people to be called in an emergency. If you're alone with your loved one, it's better to call an ambulance to go to the ER rather than drive by yourself with someone who is confused and agitated; stress can make it dangerous for both of you. Hospitals have different ER policies and you never know where you may be or what the situation might be. Chances are you will never have to visit the ER but it doesn't hurt to prepare, just in case, to make things a little easier.

There are countless reasons one goes to the ER, so remain flexible enough to be able to react to unexpected problems. It helps if the patient has something like an emergency medical bracelet indicating Alzheimer's. Much depends on whether or not someone is in mid-to-late-stage Alzheimer's, and it is critical that staff be told about Alzheimer's.

Staff will record vital signs to determine the urgency of the situation and how quickly care will be given. Again, it is imperative that you mention the patient has Alzheimer's. Sometimes they cleverly hide their dementia. Remember you are the patient's advocate and in charge. You may have to wait a bit; staff may be involved with another patient with a more serious event, be patient and reassuring.

Stay with your loved one as much as possible. ER's can be intimidating and disorienting to someone with dementia. Many questions will be asked and the patient may be unable to answer clearly, and your loved one will be touched many times by different strangers, all adding to stress. Tell each new person who sees the patient about the Alzheimer's.

At discharge, listen to the physician's discharge instructions. The patient will likely forget or misunderstand. Read and understand any discharge papers before you leave. Ask questions if you need clarification. If you need it, hospitals have social workers with information about resources after the visit, like a visiting nurse or geriatric care manager.

I had occasion to take my 90 year-old sister to the ER a few times, and she did not have dementia. But the hospital setting is very confusing and as so often happens with the elderly, she became quite difficult, not knowing where she was, what was happening and saying bizarre things. For someone with Alzheimer's, it can be even worse. So be prepared.

THE EVIL TWIN

Your Alzheimer's loved one may look the same, sound the same, move and dress the same, but inside it's someone else you've really never met. It's time to be introduced to the evil twin.

We come into this world with our own basic personality—who knows how it develops?—certainly not me. Happy, quiet, alert, somber—I've seen all types of infants grow, become adults, and most remain about the same—happy, quiet, alert, somber. Society has pressures and parents try to mould an artistic son into a sports jock; a little girl fascinated by crawling bugs is dragged to ballet lessons in a tutu. A home is loving and calm or it's a den of anger and division. Certainly upbringing and all the events in life will have an influence—and then there are things like Alzheimer's.

I think I was born a Pollyanna—annoying as that may be—I'm the peacemaker, the excuser, the naïve—well, unless you go too far and then, as my daughter says, I attack. I married a quiet man, protective; we would have a tranquil life—I expected nothing else. So, how in the hell, decades later, did he stand in front of me seething beet red, eyes bulging, veins throbbing, fists clenched screaming, "I could kill you!"

I was so stunned, I stood mute and motionless, probably the wisest thing I could have done. And then, like a violent squall it was suddenly over, quickly forgotten by him, but a life-time memory for me. My sweet love was replaced by his evil twin. I knew it was the disease that had been progressing slowly for some years, but mostly he was just about as he'd always been. Back then, I really didn't know what the biological changes were doing to his brain. In the beginning I thought

I'd just remind him of things, but it wasn't like that at all. It was something that one could not see or even understand like a rash or a cancer. But there it was, hidden, silent, inside the brain of this brilliant, loving, healthy man I'd given my life to.

So I learned that Alzheimer's is a progressive brain cell failure, and no one yet knows any reason why it happens, how to prevent it or stop it. As it destroys brain cells, it causes problems with memory, thinking and behavior severe enough to affect work, hobbies, relationships, social life, daily living routines and more. It gets worse over time and is fatal.

Our brains have 100 billion nerve cells. Each cell communicates with many others that form networks. These networks have special jobs. Some are involved in thinking, learning and remembering. Others help us see, hear and smell or tell our muscles when to move. Without our thinking about it, they control our breathing, swallowing saliva, blinking, circulation, heart beat, everything that goes on in our body.

All of these messages being sent and received are influenced by our genetics and our experiences—creating our personal essence. When cells remain healthy, we are the gentle mother, the loving husband, but when they begin to die, the messages being sent throughout the various networks become garbled; they short-circuit just as a frayed wire will mess with a lamp. And that is when the evil twin appears.

Sometimes the evil twin becomes too dangerous to live with safely. Tragically, it happened to my husband and he had to be placed. One day he went completely berserk at the facility. He ran after people, biting and hitting them, twisting arms, throwing furniture, frightening everyone and the police had to be called; he was taken to a lock-down mental facility in handcuffs. A few weeks of medication therapy calmed him back down. Years later, I still write this with a heavy heart because I know it was not really him. He was a complete stranger, no one I knew or had ever met. And, yet, his body was the same, his voice and movements—but he was being controlled by his now defective brain cells misfiring, shooting off into nowhere, not being received, missing targets, turning him into his evil twin.

This does not happen to all Alzheimer's sufferers, not at all. Some remain very placid, easy to care for, still others go into a variety of different modes that can be very difficult to deal with. The thing that is so hard to get your head around—is that they really cannot help what they are doing. There is very little logic you can use to get them to behave; they cannot compute your words. It is up to the caregiver and family to understand that they have to be the ones to change, to make the concessions, to agree even when they know something is wrong—learn not to argue, explain or try to reason. You will think some of this advice is counterintuitive, it is—but it can work.

WHAT YOU NEED TO KNOW

When brain cells are being destroyed by Alzheimer's, they alter the very essence of your loved one. There will be changes that will make you wonder, 'who is this person?' Some stay sweet and calm, but many will have their personalities become unbelievably different, even violent. Their taste buds change, their vision, their hygiene—and you will challenge them, direct them in the right way, try to drag them back to reality. Most of your efforts will fail because you cannot control the destruction of brain cells—that is inexorable.

However, once you understand the nature of the brain's destruction, there are fundamental principles you can employ to make life a bit easier for all. When there has been hostility and abuse before the disease set in, it can be devilishly difficult to love your loved one. But, inasmuch as possible, try **Love** and definitely be **Kind**. Some hints:

- ♥ What works for one Alzheimer's patient is no guarantee it will work for another.
- ♥ Practice patience, backing off, being embarrassed and keeping quiet.
- ♥ Forget logic, reasoning and fighting back.
- ♥ Don't keep explaining your mother died years ago, **lie** and say, 'She's at the market. We'll see her tomorrow." Such **lies** are a *kindness*.
- ♥ Don't ask, 'Do you want breakfast now?' Instead *announce*, 'Breakfast is ready.' Answering questions confuses those with Alzheimer's.
- ♥ Understand 'no' can mean 'yes,' 'you' can mean 'me,' and 'he' can mean 'her.'
- ♥ Agree, no matter how outrageous the situation, stay flexible.

- ♥ Apologize for whatever upsets your loved one, especially when it is **not** your fault.
- ♥ Remember to care for yourself, don't strain—keep your back strong.
- ♥ Don't be a martyr—it's highly overrated and, besides, it can kill you. Take all the help you can get.
- ♥ Choose your battles, don't sweat the small stuff, keep focused.
- ♥ Knock off the guilt, it impedes your ability to function clearly, none of it is your fault.
- ♥ A promise to care for someone doesn't mean you have to do it all alone in your own home. Sometimes professional care is best for everyone and still **fulfills** your promise.
- ♥ Stick to a daily routine *sequentially* as much as possible. Time means nothing to your loved one, sequencing is more important than timing.
- ♥ Prepare to set aside your own preferences, friends and activities.
- ♥ Be ready to rearrange your house and the schedules of all family members.
- ♥ Get rid of all guns—no excuses.
- ♥ When a loved one won't do what you want, walk away for a few minutes, come back, try again. They need time to process your words and maybe they'll never get it.
- ♥ Give instructions simply and slowly, over and over, word for word in the same tone. Changing the words changes the message and is confusing.
- ♥ When loved ones get angry, leave them alone, they're frustrated, unable to understand what's happening. Don't escalate their frustration by arguing.
- ♥ What worked on Monday may not work on Tuesday.
- ♥ *There will be times when **nothing** will work.*
- ♥ When you do everything for a loved one and they turn on you, it's hard not to take it personally.
- ♥ Don't forget face-to-face support groups, on-line message boards and chat rooms. Remember **YOU ARE NOT ALONE.** Millions of others share your woe, sorrow and travail. Reach out. Support and understanding are available.

♥ You're human—when you make mistakes, lose your temper and have bad thoughts—be **grateful** that you're normal.

♥ Cry—it cleanses your system, releases tension, and you've earned it.

♥ Laugh—really it's OK—sometimes things are just so darn funny.

Caregivers need a long time to understand and learn these things. Don't despair; no one ever gets everything right all the time. It takes practice, experimenting, trial and error, adapting and making it your own, incredible patience, and not being hard on yourself. The disease teaches you as you go along.

"There are only four kinds of people in this world:
Those who are caregivers,
Those who were caregivers,
Those who will be caregivers,
And those who will need the help of a caregiver."

Former First Lady Rosalynn Carter

GIFT IDEAS

You know, I am not sure how everyone feels about gifts. I have lived in my house over fifty years, and by now I have just about everything I'll ever need or want—I probably have two or three of *everything* and a closet full of clothes from when I was working, younger and thiiinnnnner. It was hard to get my mother a gift. Either she didn't like it (most of the time) or she put it away to 'save for good.' After she died, we found things still in their gift boxes that she'd never used. 'Good' never came. I don't want to be like that, but darn, too often I am.

I try to keep a list of things I'd, otherwise, get for myself to let my kids buy me as gifts. Last Christmas I really needed new windshield wipers and told them outright that's what I wanted. I wanted to avoid the hassle of getting them on my own. Didn't get 'em! I gave my son car tires, my daughter-in-law a laundry hamper and an attic fan for my daughter's new house. They were all thrilled, and why not? That's what they said they wanted. Bah, humbug! I still need wipers.

Such golden problems are magnified when Alzheimer's and dementia are involved. Most people mean well when they say or do things for you, but they don't always understand. My husband would get subscriptions to magazines he showed no interest in and couldn't read anyway; or tickets to a play that he wouldn't be able to follow and sit through for two hours. But they tried.

I don't have any terribly remarkable ideas and a choice of gift for someone with Alzheimer's will depend on where the recipient is at any time in the disease. Always remember to *visit, listen, accept, agree, send cards, make phone calls, visit with an appropriate pet, and give lots of hugs and kisses and then give some more.* Consider MedicAlert jewelry, 1-888-572-8566, and when appropriate, incontinence supplies.

<u>For someone in a facility:</u> Everyone has their own budget, but don't spend a lot of money. Things get lost, moved to different rooms, disappear, eaten, are thrown away, get laundered—it happens—don't sweat it. Get shoes with Velcro closures, elastic waist pants and sweat suits with tops that open in front—not over the head, calendars and books with pictures, cookies, fruit, candy, fake jewelry, wind chimes, lotions, combs and brushes, hangers, videos, music—hymns and music from their era, wallet or coin purse with an expired credit card and a little money, lap robe, warm pajamas or nightgowns, shawls, bathrobe, slippers, cuddly stuffed toy, arrange for a haircut, styling, manicure.

<u>For someone at home:</u> Much of the above and add giant button phone, simple, familiar games like checkers or dominoes, big piece jigsaw puzzles, photo album with family and friend photos, journal for people to leave messages when they visit, day-at-a-time calendar, a short car trip. Avoid board games and electronic equipment. They may be too complex and likely to frustrate rather than stimulate.

<u>And for the caregiver:</u> Time, time, time and more time. Be specific. Give a card that says, (time of your own choosing), "This card is worth the first Thursday afternoon of each month when I will take your place from one to five." Or, if you cannot do it yourself, hire a professional. Arrange for respite, housekeeping, gardening services, meals to be delivered, bring homemade meals—fresh or frozen—a carton of ice cream, certificate for dinner out, shop for groceries, pick up medications and cleaning. And, depending on the circumstances, money itself is not crass. You're bound to come up with more gift ideas yourself.

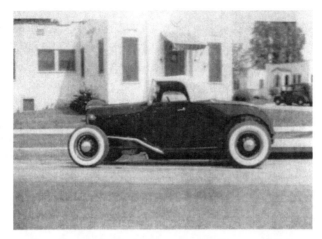

". . . he took me to the movies in a roadster
that he'd built himself."

WHEN DID YOU FIRST KNOW?

People are more than skeptical when I say that my husband had Alzheimer's from the very beginning. I fell in love with an edgy, lanky young man, a precursor to *The Fonz.* He rode a motorcycle, wore a black leather jacket and jeans that clung dangerously low to his hips, his hair was combed in a ducktail, and he took me to the movies in a roadster that he'd built himself. I liked to talk about our growing old together, when we'd both be 100, but he always countered with, "We're just a couple of punk kids."

We married in 1950 and the night before our wedding, he arrived with the ducktail gone and a flattop in its place. He was so pleased that he'd gone to a fancy hair stylist, I was stunned. Couldn't it be put back! A few weeks earlier he'd sold the roadster and bought a new, rather conventional coupe—at least it was black with whitewalls! When I asked him why, he said he couldn't drive his wife around in a roadster. But I was the same girl, wife or not, I liked the roadster. The motorcycle never came with him, it stayed at his mother's until it was sold. He never again wore the black leather jacket, jeans gave way to pleated slacks. I didn't know it then, but I now know that it was an early sign of Alzheimer's, a complete reversal of the outward manifestations of his personality. Yes, of course, people change when they marry, but not so completely—not overnight!

It didn't matter all that much, anyway, because within months he was drafted and went to Korea. When he came back, he'd again changed. Much of his spontaneous joy was gone and he kept pulling down window shades and locking doors. Yes, again, war changes a person, but he never saw battle, he was always behind the lines. Such subtle changes—probably no one else noticed.

Yet, too often people would say to me, 'why did he say or do that?' It would annoy me. I'd answer, 'don't ask me, ask him.' While it is true that I noticed changes and sometimes odd behaviors, it was never important. I just thought it was his way that he was occasionally quirky—and I loved him. It was only after decades of living with Alzheimer's and all the research, that I saw things in the past with a much different eye.

And then there was the call, when he was 24, from his supervisor at work who phoned me at home. He said that my husband didn't seem to respond to things in a normal way, that I should take him to a doctor. Huh! I had no idea what he was talking about. I never told my husband, never did anything. Eventually I came to realize that the man likely knew someone close to him who had acted the same way as my husband, he knew something was wrong. In those days, no one had yet heard the word 'Alzheimer's.' He was trying to warn me, but of what? Even he didn't know exactly.

And did my husband know? Sometimes I'd see such fear in his eyes; I'd wonder what could he be afraid of? He was by nature a brave man, but, yes, I came to believe he thought

165

he might be losing his mind and I knew him well enough to know that he'd never share such a horror with me, he'd cover it up.

And that's the way it was with my husband until the bizarre behaviors came flashing out when he was only 53 and society finally caught up with the disease. The Alzheimer's Association just revised the Ten Warning Signs of Alzheimer's disease, listed below. I appreciate that many people devoted endless hours on what is all but an impossible task. It's better, but not there yet, the disease is still too elusive, impossible for the average person to clearly 'see' it in its early stages—impossible.

(1) Memory changes that disrupt daily life, (2) Challenges in planning or solving problems, (3) Difficulty completing familiar tasks, (4) Confusion with time or space, (5) Trouble understanding visual images and spatial relationships, (6) New problems with words while speaking or writing, (7) Misplacing things and losing the ability to retrace steps, (8) Decreased or poor judgment, (9) Withdrawal from work or social activities, (10) Changes in mood or personality.

In my husband's case, I'd say (10) was the tip off, but who knew? The rest came later. I wish Alzheimer's would not be called a 'disease of forgetting.' Technically, it is forgetting, but it's so much more than that and it frightens people who all forget things on occasion. As children we don't worry about forgetting, but when older, we think, 'I'm getting Alzheimer's.' Remember, just because you forget something, especially if you later remember that you forgot, chances are that you are not getting Alzheimer's.

LINGERING EMOTIONS

There is a gentle story that routinely makes the Alzheimer's rounds. How true it is, I have no idea, but it always bears telling again. It is early morning; an elderly gentleman is at the doctor's office having a nurse remove stitches from his hand. He keeps looking at his watch, obviously anxious to leave. Idly, the nurse inquires why he's in such a hurry and he tells her that he has a 9:00 appointment to eat breakfast with his wife every day at her nursing home. The nurse wants to know if his wife will be upset if he's a few minutes late. He explains that she has Alzheimer's and hasn't known him for some time. Surprised, she says you go every morning to see her and she doesn't even know who you are. He smiles, *"She doesn't know me, but I still know who she is."*

Lingering emotions. We all have them. They take their place in our lives, sometimes buried and stored away from our daily routine for long periods of time, but they don't ever leave completely. And what about our loved ones with memory loss? Are their emotions still lingering behind those blank stares? I tend to think they are, and I'm not even sure that's such a good thing, but I think it's accurate. I will confess that I did not always consider my husband's emotions as the years of caregiving wore on. How often can it be said that I wish I knew then what I know now. That I loved him that I would protect him and care for him was a given, but, we can get so caught up in the doing of caregiving that our emotions of sadness, fear, anger, frustration, disappointment and more loom large.

Recently, researchers at the University of Iowa did a study that found that people with memory loss still 'remember' feelings associated with happy and sad experiences. I agree.

My husband did not always know who I was, how I fit into his life, but when I'd visit him in his care facility, his face would light up. I felt he knew that I was love and comfort for him, lingering emotions still very close to the surface. Of course, I'd see his face light up the same way when one of the nurses would approach him—more attention and comfort—but it was OK with me. He had positive emotions and it didn't matter where they came from, I was just happy to see him enjoy the moment.

University researchers showed happy and sad movie clips to patients with memory loss. They couldn't remember what they watched, but they did retain the emotions that were triggered by what they saw. I clearly remember my husband's coming to me if he'd seen something unpleasant on TV, emotionally distressed that we may be in danger, while something funny would leave him in a good mood. I learned to monitor his TV viewing and taped several programs I could play for him to keep him upbeat. Mr. Rogers was one of his favorites, and each tape replayed was new for him.

Lead author of the research study, Justin Feinstein, a student in the graduate programs of neuroscience and psychology, said that, "With healthy people, you see feelings decay as time goes on. In two patients, the feelings didn't decay, in fact, their sadness lingered. Sadness tended to last a bit longer than happiness, but both emotions lasted well beyond the patient's memory of the films." That seems about right to me. I tend to remember sad or negative things more frequently, and while I also remember the happy things, they do not seem to be so profound—and I am by nature a happy person.

Feinstein continued, "A simple visit or phone call from family members might have a lingering positive influence on a patient's happiness even though the patient may quickly forget the visit or phone call. On the other hand, routine neglect from staff at nursing homes may leave the patient feeling sad, frustrated and lonely even though the patient can't remember why."

It doesn't seem like much effort or imposition to make someone happy—a brief phone call, a visit with some cookies, just an 'I was thinking about you,' moment of your time. Those of you still caregiving for someone with memory problems have likely noticed the things I saw with my husband. I am certain now that as memory fades, emotions linger. I'm grateful that I eventually realized that and was able, as much as possible, to keep sadness and fear at bay and encourage any small moments of happiness for him.

CHANGES IN THE FIVE SENSES

SMELL, TASTE, SIGHT, TOUCH, HEARING

(1) SMELL & TASTE

It has been demonstrated that a fetus can feel pain and hear, so our senses are working even before we are born. Normally, if we smell smoke, we look for fire (smell); spit out bad tasting food (taste); shift our eyes when driving (sight); flinch from a hot stove (touch); and adjust the TV volume (hearing). It is constant and never ending. We can understand the tragedy and danger involved for those who are blind or deaf or even if they cannot smell. My Mother broke her nose on a swing set as a young girl and after two botched surgeries was left unable to smell. She could not smell perfume, escaping gas or if something was burning on the stove, maybe that's why our food never burned; she carefully watched everything she cooked.

Because our brains are so programmed, our body reacts 24/7 to things we never consciously tell it to do. Blood circulates, food digests and is eliminated, eyes blink, saliva is swallowed, hearts beat, lungs fill with air, livers detoxify—busy, busy, busy activity. Unless it is something unusual like what happened to my Mother, it doesn't seem possible that someone can't smell properly. But with Alzheimer's, as brain cells are damaged—*and you cannot see that it is happening*—senses can go haywire.

While smell may diminish in some healthy elderly people, research has shown that those with early stages of cogitative impairment have trouble identifying common odors like baby powder, natural gas, lemon, chocolate, fish, smoke. It can be an early indication of which people will go on to develop

Alzheimer's, and when they do, the deficit increases as the disease progresses. If you don't already have one in the house, it's a good idea to get a working smoke detector.

Smell seems to be affected before other senses in Alzheimer's and, knowing this, can help with earlier awareness and medications. Eventually, it may happen that, unlike an expensive brain scan, a specifically designed smell test will be a cheaper way to make an early diagnosis.

Obviously smell goes along with taste, and again, taste can decline with age in the healthy. My husband never had a sweet tooth, but he developed one with Alzheimer's. Others have complained that food is tasteless, like having a bad cold. Also, smoking, poor oral care and loss of smell can make food taste unpleasant and could cause loss of appetite and someone to stop eating altogether. People who ate bland foods before may now insist on lots of salt, sugar and other spicy seasonings; or they forget that they just ate and what specific foods smell and taste like.

Along with loss of smell and taste sensitivity, and as judgment declines, those with Alzheimer's may place dangerous or inappropriate things in their mouths. Keep an eye on the possibility of their using excessive amounts of condiments; be careful of things like toothpaste, medicines, rubbing alcohol, and soap that may look and smell like food; clean old and spoiled food out of the refrigerator that may cause food poisoning if consumed, and lock it if necessary. Keep pet litter boxes out of sight and be watchful if you store pet food in the refrigerator; do your best to see that dentures fit properly and keep an extra set, if possible. Check drawers and other hiding places for food hoarding. If you think something dangerous has been eaten, call the poison control center (1-800-222-1222) or 911 immediately. Consider that many people eat better when socializing so try to eat together and avoid distractions like the TV.

It's a personal issue, but depending on the stage your loved one is in, I never worried too much about my husband's overall health and what he ate. It is not uncommon for Alzheimer's patients to lose weight, no matter how well they eat and it's not like they are children who absolutely need essential nutrients for their growth and future health. It's one of very few pleasures left to them, so forget the veggies, go for the chocolate sundae with whipped cream, nuts and a cherry on top!

CHANGES IN THE FIVE SENSES

SMELL, TASTE, SIGHT, TOUCH, HEARING
(2) SIGHT

Standing next to each other, my husband showed me his house key resting on his open palm. He had no idea what it was. In simple analogy, my normal eyes took a photo of the key, the image went to the brain cells that control sight and they did their job developing the mental picture necessary to tell me what I saw. My husband's normal eyes took a photo of the key, the image went to the brain cells that control sight but they were so damaged and out of whack that they could not develop the mental picture necessary to tell him what he saw. This is also part of not recognizing familiar faces; it's not just a matter of forgetting who a person is. Often, once people are identified, they are remembered.

Early symptoms of visual problems may be asking to see the eye doctor but there will be no changes in the eyes and no problems with prescriptions. There may be under or over reaching for objects; grabbing the car's side mirror, instead of the door handle; driving too close or too far from the car in front; tripping on familiar ground and making missteps; falling when going up or down stairs. You can avoid some of this if you put bright tape or paint on the stair edges for contrast. These are indications that the sense of perception, depth and color may all be changing.

A woman will be unable to step into a white tile shower because she cannot distinguish between the white tile bathroom floor and where the white tile shower floor begins. She will 'see' the difference if you put a colored bath rug on the floor next to the shower.

Those with Alzheimer's often need ***contrast*** to 'see' something, so do not put mashed potatoes on a white plate or tomatoes on a red one. There are inexpensive colorful plastic dishes you can buy and you may have to use several for any given meal, but it will be more appetizing, help them 'see' their food and eat better. If they are bumping into furniture—maybe a table is the same color as the carpet—put a contrasting color tablecloth on the table, a throw or a sheet on a couch. Even a small sleeping pet that is the same color as the floor can cause someone to trip. Bright large bows on a collar or a pet sweater can help. Keep things well lit and offer guidance in dim areas.

Be careful with holiday decorations. A Christmas tree and lots of decorations that suddenly appear in the home can be confusing and disturbing, and Halloween or Mardi Gras masks can be frightening when Alzheimer's patients have trouble distinguishing between a mask and a real face. They may see a dark rug as a hole in the ground and step around it, or on a big white and black checkerboard floor, they'll only step on the white tiles. On the other hand, if you put a mural of trees or bookshelves on a door, they will no longer see it as a door and that can help keep them from going outside and wandering. Such murals are available at wallpaper websites and stores.

All sorts of strange things happen when the brain alters what the eye sees. Riding in the passenger seat of a car, a man with Alzheimer's may flinch as he perceives objects outside coming at him. You can see how dangerous it would be to drive. Someone may be perfectly able to operate the mechanics of a car, but can he judge the speed of a train coming from the side at a railroad crossing?

From time to time we all see reflections in dark windows or figures in clouds, shadows in trees. But those with Alzheimer's can think they are real, so drawing curtains at night and covering or removing some mirrors will help avoid that. My husband could not recognize himself in the mirror, and he often had a good conversation with that 'nice man.' It was difficult for me to watch at first, but since he seemed to enjoy the visits, I let it be. He also had many pleasant discussions with a large figurine of a dog that sat on the floor near our couch. Sadly, he came to live in his own reality. It was easier for both of us if I did not try to change that.

CHANGES IN THE FIVE SENSES

SMELL, TASTE, SIGHT, TOUCH, HEARING

(3) TOUCH
BODY TEMPERATURE &
THERAPEUTIC TOUCH

Those with Alzheimer's may no longer be able to interpret feelings of cold, heat or discomfort as the cells in the section of the brain that regulate body temperature become damaged, and they may shiver and complain of being overly cold when everyone else is comfortable. Normally we are aware of pressure, vibration, temperature, pain, and where we are touched, but that sense, like the others, can also diminish with age so there could be more than one cause in play since many with Alzheimer's are already elderly. There are any number of reasons why someone may be excessively cold; anemia, thyroid, circulation, weight loss, nutritional deficiencies like iron, and loss of the fatty cushion in the thinning skin of the elderly. It is important, then, if this continues to see a physician, it may be something easily remedied.

I knew a man with Alzheimer's who was always so cold that his family had a dedicated room in the house that they kept heated for him all year long, even in the summers. In spite of that, he needed to be bundled up with sweaters, jackets, hats and gloves—and still said he was cold.

Stories abound of those with Alzheimer's going out in the snow with a t-shirt and shorts, they cannot express why they feel hot or cold, so it is up to the caregiver to determine if it is indeed hot or cold and help them dress and behave appropriately. The caregiver should be as supportive as possible and validate any concerns. It doesn't pay to argue the point or show them the thermostat; they will believe what they believe. When they think they are hot and undress, it can be more difficult, so try cool drinks, ice cream, a small electric fan and the usual distractions.

If you can't have a separate room, remember that others have to live in the house, too. If someone is cold, try warming clothes in the dryer, a small electric heater just for a specific area, having a supply of socks, slippers, robes and blankets may do the trick without having to overheat the entire house, and have goodies like hot chocolate, hot-grilled sandwiches, soup, tea, hot toddy, if you're so inclined.

You can lower your hot water temperature to avoid accidental scalding. Signs like 'very hot,' or 'do not touch,' on the oven, coffee maker, toaster, iron and other such appliances may help, and unplug them when not in use. Check shower and bath water temperature before bathing, and be careful offering food that's too hot.

Touch is an important means of communicating. Residents may be deprived of touch in care facilities, so take extra time and effort for appropriate physical contact to offer affection, love, safety and security.

I have no knowledge of whether 'touch' is universal or cultural, but I used to be a docent at the zoo and over and over you will see animals naturally hug, cuddle, touch, slap, pet and roll around together. In some cultures men hug, in others it is not acceptable; in some, women hold hands, walk arm-in-arm, in others they do not. I've been with some families where the hugging and kissing—both cheeks—hello and goodbye can take half a day, while others wave a cheery 'see ya' and are out the door.

The deeper my husband went into Alzheimer's, the more I needed to touch him for myself and to let him know I was there. I'd visit the care facility with cookies we'd share sitting thigh to thigh on a sofa, my head on his shoulder, or if he was asleep on his bed, I'd curl up at his back, spoon fashion, just to feel his familiar warmth and hear his breathing. I know it's not for everyone, but what is more intimate, more loving than a connecting touch.

CHANGES IN THE FIVE SENSES

SMELL, TASTE, SIGHT, TOUCH, HEARING

(4) HEARING

I would stand behind my husband, speak clearly into his ear and he would not respond. I could have been a feather falling; he was simply unable to put it all together. When the ear hears the sound of a spoken word, the brain has to process its meaning—but Alzheimer's can get it all bollixed up because of damage to the brain cells. Those with this disease do not follow conversations well or simple requests and may correctly process only parts of a sentence—words and sounds. If I asked my husband to water the plants on the patio, he did not process 'the plants,' but he'd process 'patio,' so he watered the patio bricks.

With hearing problems, the misunderstandings intensify. Certainly hearing can be tested, but hearing aides will not fix brain damage, although if needed, they can help. They are, however, often expensive, easily lost and confusing for the Alzheimer's patient to wear.

When speaking to your loved one, repeating doesn't always help the processing. Rephrase your words into shorter, simpler sentences. If there is also a hearing problem, speak louder (don't shout), more slowly and look directly at the person. Instead of saying, 'get dressed,' you might break it down to, 'put on your slacks,' then 'put on your shirt,' then 'socks,' then 'shoes.'

Like many others, I do not hear well with background noise, conversation and music—and it has to be harder for someone with Alzheimer's; avoid excessive noise in the house, like

stereo both on; be sensitive to noise outside
windows and doors if necessary; avoid large
ple if your loved one shows signs of distress
rowds; keep away from screaming, laughing
eone has a hearing aid, check the batteries
and   frequently.

Our senses: Smell, Taste, Sight, Touch and Hearing are designed to protect us. We hear a loud noise—we are instantly alert—adrenalin starts pumping; the sun burns our skin, we seek shade; we see a stranger lurking, we consider flight. When these vital senses diminish with age or become scrambled because of brain damage we are at an increased risk of injury. Think of how frightened and vulnerable Alzheimer's patients must feel. No wonder they fear being left alone and cling to their caregiver, the one person who is their protector.

This places on-going burdens on caregivers. Not only do you have to think and remember for your loved one, sometimes you even have to see and hear for them. It can be hard, if not impossible, for at-home caregivers to get help and, to be honest, more often than not, the caregiver will not seek help or even refuse it when offered. It cannot be said enough: The caregiver's life and health is just as important as the person with Alzheimer's. Please, if you are a caregiver, take care of yourself, you're worth it.

RONALD REAGAN

Politics aside, this is about one person who had Alzheimer's. It is well to remember that the disease does not discriminate—Democrat or Republican, rich or poor, active or sedentary, educated or unschooled, famous or obscure, every race, every religion, atheists. What we can learn from each other about this disease as individuals and families trumps everything else.

Because it took me a long time before I overcame an emotional barrier about my husband's Alzheimer's and was able to speak honestly and publicly about it, I understand the profound sacrifice of personal privacy and dignity it took for Reagan to write his poignant 1994 letter announcing his illness. He wrote: *Upon learning this news, Nancy & I had to decide whether as private citizens we would keep this a private matter or whether we would make the news known in a public way . . . now, we feel it is important to share it with you. In opening our hearts, we hope this might promote greater awareness of this condition. Perhaps it will encourage a clearer understanding of the individuals and families who are affected by it.*

Both our families were going through this scourge at the same time. I did not have to hear any updates about the Reagan's. Nancy, no doubt, had an abundance of help, but like everyone with an Alzheimer's loved one, she and their children still lived in a world of hurt and horror. His decision to go public greatly affected society's perception of Alzheimer's and reducing its stigma, although for far too many, that stigma still looms.

In 1995, the Reagan's founded the **Ronald and Nancy Reagan Research Institute,** an affiliate of the National Alzheimer's

Association in Chicago. The institute marked an important milestone in Alzheimer's research as it largely introduced and expanded the biological segment of disease research with a focus on a commitment to innovative cutting-edge basic science for exploring the broadest possible approaches to developing treatments for Alzheimer's.

Later, Nancy would devote her time to supporting federally-funded **embryonic** stem cell research hoping it would lead to an Alzheimer's cure. Just recently a court lifted the ban on federal funding of embryonic stem cell research. *(As a layman, I don't think that will be effective for helping Alzheimer's. If I had that kind of money, I'd use it to research DNA. We know that a minority of cases is genetic and I think, as with my husband, that Alzheimer's is likely caused by a recessive gene. I do, however, support **adult** stem cell research.)*

Until her death in 2001, Reagan's daughter Maureen was very active in the Reagan Institute. In 1999 she was appointed a member of the Alzheimer's Association's National Board and served as the group's spokeswoman raising awareness of the disease and especially support for caregivers, saying, "There's a special place in heaven for caregivers," after watching Nancy care for her father. She is credited with raising sixty million dollars for Alzheimer's research.

Daughter Patti has written about Alzheimer's and her father in her book, *The Long Goodbye.* I have only read reviews and excerpts, but they tell me that she nails the way the disease destroys not only the victim's life, but profoundly effects the lives of others. She writes, "Alzheimer's snips away at the threads, a slow unraveling, a steady retreat; as a witness all you can do is watch, cry, and whisper a soft stream of goodbyes." And, that's exactly how it happens.

In an on-going effort to educate the public about Alzheimer's, Reagan's son Michael is also Chairman of the Board of Directors of *The John Douglas French Alzheimer's Foundation.* Since 2004 I have been an Honorary Member of the Foundation whose mission is to serve as a venture catalyst to provide critical seed money to major California universities for novel and promising Alzheimer's research, generally not funded by the government or pharmaceuticals.

As for son Ron's writing in his book, *My Father at 100,* that Reagan had Alzheimer's while he was President—it's likely to remain an unresolved issue. I know that over the years my husband would say or do something that I attributed to distraction, fatigue, depression—whatever. Later I came to believe much of it was the unrecognized onset of the disease—or maybe it *was* simply distraction and fatigue—there's no telling—and either way, he still functioned just fine.

I'm not sure that Reagan's falling asleep during cabinet meetings was an early indication of Alzheimer's. Maybe he was just tired and bored. People fall asleep at speeches, concerts, school, the movies. At times we all misspeak, president or not, and it's normal to forget things on occasion, it's part of the human condition and rarely a precursor to Alzheimer's.

Nancy writes in her book, *I Love You Ronnie,* that she initially did not see signs of illness—and who would know better than a spouse? But then there is denial and I swam in that river for a long time. Although my husband's behavior sometimes caused friction between us, occasional tiffs happen in every family—maybe he simply *was* annoyed with me at the moment.

I do know that someone is not just fine one day and diagnosed with Alzheimer's the next. It comes on over a period of many years, even decades, and during those times the person is quite capable and self-reliant, holding down a job, making responsible decisions, participating properly in all aspects of every day life until unexplained events send someone to a doctor. Most people are stunned by the diagnosis—they think 'not him, he's too intelligent, too active, too healthy, it has to be a misdiagnosis'—and sometimes it is—it's not always easy to diagnose accurately.

In my view, the hand-written Alzheimer's letter Reagan wrote five years after leaving office shows that the handwriting is firm and legible, the grammar is correct, there's no rambling, nothing to indicate to the casual observer that anything is wrong, although those qualities deteriorate as the illness progresses. He knew he had the disease on that day, but it would be some time before his thought processes and capabilities slipped entirely away. Admirers and detractors will never stop fussing about it. Might just as well let it be, there are no mulligans for history.

(For a list of the many prominent people who have had Alzheimer's disease or have someone in their family with the condition, please visit: www.caregiving4alz.com, and scroll down to 'You're In Good Company.')

DIAGNOSING ALZHEIMER'S AND DEMENTIA

Alzheimer's disease and dementia often confuse people. **Alzheimer's** is a disease like cancer, diabetes, polio, lupus, heart disease, multiple sclerosis, or Huntington's. However, it is not contagious, it cannot be prevented and no one knows what causes it.

Dementia <u>is neither a disease nor an illness.</u> It is a condition; a description of symptoms that may appear in over 70 diseases or other medical conditions. It is caused by the death of brain cells resulting in the gradual deterioration of mental functioning such as concentration, memory and judgment, and affects a person's ability to perform normal daily activities. Think of dementia as a fever. A fever may be present if you have pneumonia, appendicitis, or an infected tooth; but a <u>fever is neither a disease nor an illness,</u> it is a symptom indicating that something is wrong. You have to find out what is causing the fever or dementia. Dementia may create language problems; getting lost in familiar places; disorientation about time, people and place; neglecting personal safety, hygiene and nutrition; unable to solve simple tasks; trouble making change; mood swings; agitation; repeating things.

Most dementias occur gradually, over many years, unless it is from a stroke, accident or injury, and would then happen abruptly. It may be caused by Alzheimer's, Parkinson's, reactions to meds, infections, diminished oxygen, excessive alcohol or drug use, and much more. Some dementias, but not Alzheimer's, are reversible, so it is important to find the cause, and it is not a part of normal aging.

185

Alzheimer's disease accounts for upwards of 65% of all dementias and usually shows short-term memory loss as its first and primary symptom. **Lewy Body disease** is lesser known but still presents significant dementia; usually balance and hallucinations appear earlier than with Alzheimer's. **Vascular dementia** comes from strokes and mini-strokes with varying symptoms depending on where the stroke occurs in the brain. Sometimes there is memory loss, sometimes, not. **Frontotemporal dementia** usually shows changes in personality and lack of inhibition rather than memory problems early in the disease.

These are the four major brain disorders that cause dementia but there are many others with far fewer patients. At this time, there are no medicines to cure or prevent them. Some dementias, like those that come from something like B-12 deficiency, thyroid imbalance, hormonal disorder or hydrocephalus (water on the brain) are treatable. So it is important to get a valid diagnosis when dementia occurs, and therein, lays the problem for many.

You can easily see how these symptoms of dementia overlap from one condition to another. Types of dementia are not always easy to assess. Diagnosis is made by taking a patient's medical history and doing a complete physical and neurological exam. The doctor will interview those close to the patient to determine mental functioning and use tests such as asking the patient to recall words, list of objects and recent events. Blood tests, PET and CT scans can help determine the cause of the dementia, and just as importantly, to rule out other things that may be causing the dementia, such as a tumor.

At *Lunds universitet* in Sweden, a study was done on 176 patients who had all been examined at specialist geriatric psychiatry clinics from 1996 to 2006 and diagnosed with some form of dementia. At autopsy, their brains were studied under a microscope and researchers were able to precisely establish which type of dementia the patients had.

In 49% of cases the clinical diagnosis agreed w autopsy; 14% the diagnosis was partly in agreement; in 37% an entirely different diagnosis was made after t patient's death. The highest level of correct diagnoses was in patients with frontotemporal dementia, the accuracy of the diagnoses was somewhat lower for those with Alzheimer's, vascular dementia or Lewy Body dementia.

Currently, no diagnosis of Alzheimer's is 100% accurate. However, using the latest advanced methods, a qualified physician can come close to being 90% accurate. Most doctors do their best, but the science of complete accuracy is not there yet. For the moment it cannot be helped, some people will be misdiagnosed. Still, if you feel you or a loved one has not had an accurate diagnosis, get a second or third opinion. Typically, dementia lasts about seven years after diagnosis, but it can last for as much as twenty, so it is worth any effort to get the best diagnosis available.

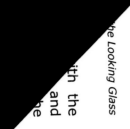

E FALLEN AND I CAN'T GET UP."

I did, I fell and I couldn't get up. I slipped in semi-darkness on a bottom step that I'd been on a thousand times and went down on a concrete path. Fortunately my head hit a border shrub, my left palm was bruised from breaking my fall, but my lower legs took the brunt of it. Left shin and outside ankle bone were bruised and swollen, inside right knee also deeply bruised and swollen, making walking difficult—I was gimpy for some time.

But I could not get up. True, my legs are aging, but it was more than that. I needed to sit where I was for a bit, to regain myself. I wouldn't let people lift me until I was ready, and then it was five or six days before I felt that my body had re-set. In the movies, people run, fall down, get right back up and continue running. That wasn't the way it happened to me.

Two things came of the event: (1) I fell on concrete and nothing broke! I must have good bones for my age. (2) Maybe I should think about buying one of those emergency call buttons to wear, because I know if it happens again and I'm alone, I won't be able to get up—and strong bones or not, something might break. When I fell, everyone was concerned and not too surprised because of my age; but there was nothing unique about it, people fall—young or old—sick or well.

Alzheimer's patients present special problems when they fall, and one of the best things caregivers can do is to try to prevent them as much as possible, because those with this disease have a high risk of falling. They have difficulty walking, balance becomes impaired, eyesight and depth perception change,

they are confused navigating around furniture, '
from bed to chair or just standing up.

You can start by checking your house for sharp edges on tables and furniture that moves when leaned on. Keep walkways clear of toys, wiring and clutter, have adequate lighting. Throw rugs should be removed or securely taped down. Consider putting a colorful bow on small pets so they are easily seen. Wipe up spills immediately. Keep walking aids close to your loved one's bed and things they use near their chair or on shelves within easy reach.

Stairs should be well lit, have handrails on both sides and grab bars for tricky places. Put white or bright yellow tape on step edges so they know where the edge is. If needed, consider a child's gate at the top or bottom of any stairs. If there is carpet, check to see if it is frayed, and if you have wood floors, don't polish them. Outside steps should not be wet or slippery, keep your loved one inside until they are dry and safe.

Have grab bars at the patient's height throughout the house wherever falls might occur, especially in the bathroom. Have them in the tub/shower, near the toilet, consider a shower chair and raised toilet seat. Use a handheld shower head on a flexible hose. Don't use bath oil in a tub. Have a non-slip tub/shower mat. If the floor and shower entrance are both the same color, put a non-skid contrasting color rug outside the shower so the patient can see where to step in.

Other risk factors include hearing and vision problems, mental confusion and decreased feeling in the feet or undiagnosed foot pain; medications that reduce perception or cause dizziness; and having unrealistic expectations of their current abilities. Weak muscles and joints, decreased reaction time, alcohol use and even 'fear of falling,' especially if they've fallen before, all add to the problem.

And don't forget footwear. No flippy-floppies or backless sandals, no heels higher then 1-1/2 inches, no slippery soles, don't walk around in socks on wood or linoleum floors. Tennis shoes that lace up are good and so are Velcro closures. Don't let the shoes be so loose that the foot moves around too much or may come out. Make sure that pant legs, nightgowns and robes are not too long.

You know, you can only do so much, but a few precautions in advance may eliminate a lot of emotional and medical problems that can come with falls. You'll never really know how many falls your actions may have prevented and, if someone falls anyway, give credit to yourself that you tried.

FINDING IN-HOME HELP

I hadn't even thought about in-home help, but a neighbor across the street told me about a man who was a really good caregiver. I didn't know at some point she and my husband had become friends, that she was aware of his condition, and it wasn't long before I called the man. He was named Angel, from the Philippines; if ever an angel was heaven-sent, it was him. He knew more about Alzheimer's and what to do than I did at the time. I just let him take over and teach me. But the time came when my husband did not like another man in the house and he finally twisted Angel's arm, threatened him, and I had to let him go.

Again, the stars lined up and someone told me about Terry from Belize—another angel. My husband liked her and she liked him. She'd do anything for him until she had to leave for personal reasons. Over time I'd call agencies and they'd send me their best experienced Alzheimer's aides. Yeah, right! It was one misfit after another. Now, let me tell you what I learned along the way.

I was not prepared at all when I called the agencies. I was not specific enough about what I needed the aide to do—I didn't do any research or interview anyone—just accepted who they sent. I should have asked about their past home aide experience; what kind of training they had; why they wanted to do this type of work (it's not for everyone); why did they leave their last job; are there things they won't or can't do (is the patient incontinent, is there a wheelchair involved, will they bathe the patient); will they do cooking and light housework; do they like pets, are they allergic to a pet in the home; will they drive the loved one to appointments, run errands; do they have a car, insurance (ask to see insurance

191

proof); do they understand about Alzheimer's patients and their resistance to care; have they handled emergencies; will you need them for medical care, are they qualified to give injections, physical therapy or whatever else is required? I was home with my husband, but some people work and must leave an aide alone with a loved one—something else to think about.

If references have been given, call and ask how long the reference has known the applicant; describe what you want them to do and ask if the reference thinks they can do it; did the applicant get along well with the patient, you, and others in the home; why did they leave; and would you rehire the applicant; were they cheerful and willing to pitch in, was there any patient abuse or neglect?

Start looking for an agency by asking your doctor, hospital, senior center or care facility. Ask family, friends, church or other organization members, and co-workers. Contact your County Agency on Aging; look in the yellow pages under things like 'home care' or 'nursing.'

Now ask the agency how long they have been in business; how do they train employees; are they licensed (ask to see papers); ask about available services and fees; is there a supervisor to oversee quality of care; are they and their employee bonded; how do they handle emergencies; what about client confidentially; how do you get billed and pay for any extra fees or insurance coverage; do they have written explanations of their policies; do they accept Medicare or Medicaid; do they have references for both the agency and the prospective employee; is there a complaint procedure?

Of course you will have additions or deletions to these lists. They are only meant as a guide. I wish I'd been more aware when I was going through it. You will hear horror tales about aides and you will hear wonderful, uplifting stories as well. You may have to go through several people before you find the right fit for yourself and your loved one. But they are out there. I'll never forget Angel and Terry and am eternally grateful for the care they gave my husband, the help they gave and all they taught me.

SHADOWING & SUNDOWNING

Shadowing—My dear husband clung so close to me that I thought he might come between me and my shadow. And that's exactly what this behavior is called—'shadowing.' It drove me nuts, I told him to go away, pushed him away, all but hid from him. At the computer, he'd be breathing down my neck; when I was in the bathroom he'd knock on the door, call to me. Maybe it should be called 'smothering,' because that's what it does to the caregiver.

Good grief, I thought, give me some space, some breathing room, but it wasn't until I went for a doctor's appointment one day and left him home alone that I began to understand. He was in a panic when I came back, terrified that I'd left him, and I knew I could never leave him alone again, he had to have me in his sight at all times; I was his tether to safety.

Long before I knew he had Alzheimer's, I'd often see fear in his eyes. Why? He was a brave, strong man; he'd fight to the death for me and the children. True, we sometimes had difficult financial times, but it was more than that—we lived a safe ordinary life—it would be years before I'd learn that he knew he was losing his mind, that he had a brain disease neither one of us understood nor suspected.

The time comes when the Alzheimer's individual realizes that he has no control, nothing makes sense, things are not where they should be, familiar people are strangers, he's often lost—even in his own house. It has to be like tumbling in space, not knowing which way is up or where the earth is. So they cling to the one person who has been a constant in their life, the one they can trust to keep them safe and secure.

It will help if you speak frequent reassuring words: "You are safe, I am here, I won't let anything bad happen, I'm glad you are with me, everything is OK, I love you." Further, do not make changes in the home or daily routine; try to keep it all simple, familiar and calm. Eventually it stops.

Sundowning—If you've had a baby, you may have noticed that they often start to fuss about dinner time, the end of the day when everyone has had it. Same with Alzheimer's. Obviously it could be fatigue; they spend so much of their time trying to fit in, to understand what is happening around them, it's exhausting. Low lighting adds to their confusion, more shadows appear and sleep patterns are disrupted. Plan outdoor activities in the sunlight to encourage nighttime sleepiness. Lack of sunlight for anyone can cause people to feel depression during winter weather. Get as much sunlight as possible during the day and at night keep lots of bright lights on.

As night comes on, draw drapes so that reflections in the windows do not frighten them; keep a night light on in the bedroom and bathroom, limit caffeine and sugar to morning time; have dinner early and maybe a light bedtime snack; in an unfamiliar place, like a hospital, bring familiar items, a photo album, a small radio, their pillow, robe and slippers.

Often people have done the same thing at the same time for decades. Perhaps at 5:00 p.m., Mom has always started dinner. Now she's forgotten what she has to do. She knows it's important, people are depending on her, but she can't remember what it is. Frustration and agitation set in, she's worried, starts pacing. If it's possible, let her help with dinner, or do something domestic to make her feel useful. With Dad, he could have closed his office every day for 30 years, put away the open files, locked his desk, the windows and doors, checked that the alarm was set. He's all primed and ready to—to do what? You might give him some junk mail and ask him to open and sort it. Again, it can make him feel useful. When you understand why they exhibit these behaviors, you can think about what you can do to help them and help yourself at the same time.

I don't remember sundowning problems with my husband, but I well recall being awakened at 3:00 or 4:00 in the morning to find that he was fully dressed and ready to go to work. Getting him all reversed and back into bed was a challenge. So it wasn't at sundown, does it matter! No wonder caregivers are often sleep-deprived—and that's never good for anyone.

GUILT

When my father died, my mother was full of guilt. If only I'd done this, done that, she cried, he'd still be here. But she was a good woman, a good wife; she always took care of him and all of us. It was his time, and nothing she could have done would have changed that.

Guilt can be a very strong and too-familiar companion. Some people are so attached to their guilt that they feel guilty when it rains on your birthday. It could be upbringing, religion, the demands of society, but why do so many people waste all that emotional and mental energy on something so destructive by thinking over and over again, "If I'd only done more, if I'd only tried harder—the guilt is killing me!"? It may do that if you don't change your thoughts, you're just not that powerful. No matter how guilty you may feel, you don't have the ability to control what you can't control, no matter how hard you think you have to try. So don't keep packing your bags for another guilt trip.

Instead, say to yourself what I've repeated and repeated to myself or anyone who dares to criticize: "It's not my fault, I didn't cause this and I don't have the power to stop it. I'm proud of how I took care of him, how strong I was and how much I helped him, but I'm only human. As hard as I tried, I couldn't do what the rest of the world has been unable to do, but I did my best until my own well-being was comprised. I have nothing to feel guilty about—and I won't feel guilty and I won't let anyone lay any guilt on me. I was powerless to control this disease; I could do no more than I could reasonably do." Now, don't cop out on any of it, don't look for loopholes.

The great irony about guilt is that truly guilty people rarely feel guilty. Someone is convicted of a crime, goes to jail, comes back out and does the same thing all over again. Watch television court shows and see how many people are caught in lies, deny they wrote something, that it's their voice on a tape, their face in a video. They rarely admit guilt, even after losing the case they leave the courtroom and insist they're innocent, they were framed or it was all a big mistake.

It's time for Alzheimer's caregivers and those of you who have done nothing wrong to stop feeling guilty—stop searching for something to feel guilty about—and begin to reprogram your minds. So repeat, "I didn't do anything wrong and I refuse to keep feeling guilty!" Say it once a day, eleven times, thirty-seven, two hundred and nine, whatever it takes. Could you have done just one more thing for your loved one, just one more time? Probably, yes, but it wouldn't have made any difference, except that you'd be sick yourself. Did you have bad thoughts? Probably, yes, everyone does from time to time, but you didn't always follow through on them, did you?

<u>Not only does guilt prevent you from making decisions in your own best interest, it also prevents you from making decisions in the best interest of your loved one.</u> Sometimes your doing everything all by yourself is not the best thing for your loved one. Maybe he needs someone who is not stressed out, sleep deprived, resentful and exhausted. It's bad enough what Alzheimer's does to you, don't let guilt add to your stress, you don't need it and it won't help your loved one. There's no reason for you to carry unfounded guilt—let it go.

Too often a caregiver is not taking care of a 'loved one,' she's taking care of an angry, hostile mother who's been mean-spirited all of her life; or maybe it's an abusive father, an indifferent grandparent. You can hardly blame people if they don't volunteer for added years of increased anguish. And yet, many of them take on that role, perhaps with resentment and frustration, but they do it. Maybe guilt plays a part, maybe not, but either way they deserve a gold star for not opting out.

One more thing, be sure to tell your husband, often, how much you have always loved him and appreciate all that he did for you, how he worked so hard to support the family, taught values to the children, was there to help; tell your wife how much you always loved her, what a wonderful, comfortable, happy home she made; cared for the children and supported you when you tried new ventures. Tell your mother how well you remember the little things she did for you, how much that birthday cake meant, the dress she hemmed, how important her guidance was, the special Sunday dinners. Remind your father of the things he taught you, how to skim a rock over the lake, to drive, to use tools, to be strong and gentle. The more you do this, the more you express your personal love and appreciation, the less guilt you will feel—and somehow, somewhere, your loved one will understand and feel a warm glow inside. You won't get another chance.

OLDEST OLD

Yup, that's me on the fast track to becoming one of what is currently called the 'oldest old.' My credentials are an almanac of aches, a profusion of pains, a passel of pills; and compression stockings that may not look adorable, but honestly, once you wrestle them on, they really are quite comfortable.

I'm not fond of that 'oldest' designation—although I am happy enough to be there. Humans have given themselves all sorts of age ladders over the years; most notably Shakespeare's Seven Ages of Man. Today there's a social/economic category for those between 45 and 75 known as the 'Third Age,' and they live about 30 years longer than their forebears of 1900. That's probably most of you readers. My children are 'Third Age!' So what are we who have outlived the Third Age? Oldest old, I guess.

The youngest of three daughters, I think about my sisters and aging with good reason. A month before she died a few years ago at 90, Ruth told me about her seniors' group Poker Night. When her grey-haired, bifocaled, 4' 11" presence was seated in a waiting empty chair at the table of middle-aged powerful poker playing men, there was much moaning and muttering about having to play with some ol' broad. "And did you wipe up the floor with them?" I asked. "Oh, yeah," she chortled.

Ruth's life was the most difficult, but she faced each day with a 'take your best shot' attitude, I learned a lot from her. She got a pacemaker in her mid-80's and it did not slow her down—not one bit. She'd visit doctors younger than her grandchildren, explain to them what the problem was, give them a lesson or two, then tell me, "Betty, they just don't know what to do with us."

Lois, always considered the smart one, just turned 90. For several years she has complained about her memory, cognitively declining. It's not Alzheimer's, probably vascular. She gave me an outdated camping wall map of the United States for my recent birthday and one of her ancient faded photo albums brightly wrapped with a bow for Christmas. Oh, well. A hired woman is with her most of the time. They go shopping, to the movies, lunch, the park, visit me or others, and Lois enjoys the fussing over her, seeing that she eats properly, help to steady her walking, a jacket to put on or take off. The aim is to keep her in her home as long as possible.

With one 90 year old sister having been sharp as a tack and the other 90 year old sister sharp as a marble, I can't help looking over my shoulder. *Capiche?* I hope the odds are in my favor; according to a study done by the Women Cognitive Impairment Study of Exceptional Aging, at the University of California, San Francisco, more than 40 percent of women 85 and older have symptoms of Alzheimer's or other serious thinking and memory problems. That's what they called us, 'oldest old.' We are the fastest growing segment in the United States, and expected to increase by 40 percent in the next decade alone and I'm afraid they still don't know what to do with us.

The research followed 1,300 women 85 and up. Twenty seven percent were over 90. Forty one percent or 634 women had serious memory and thinking problems, while the remaining 665 tested normal. Most of those with dementia had Alzheimer's or a mix of Alzheimer's and vascular dementia. About 12 percent has vascular dementia alone. Mild cognitive impairment, (MCI), a serious form of memory loss that can lead to Alzheimer's was also common to the group.

Alzheimer's and other dementias almost double with every 5 years of age after 65. About 2 to 3 percent of those 65 to 75 have dementia, compared to 35 percent in those 85 and older.

MCI was higher in women over 90 than in those between 85 and 89. Most, but not all, had serious memory problems.

Such studies are critical for public health planning and for families as the population continues to age and the oldest old increase. People used to have lots of children with the idea that those who lived would take care of them when they aged. Who do people today think will care for them in their dotage? Of my 29 adult nieces and nephews, half are childless. What about your family? That much dementia in a growing elderly population plus sick or injured younger people now kept alive who would have died generations past—all requiring 24/7 major medical care—presents a difficult caring equation. I don't know of any easy answers.

WHO CARES FOR THE ELDERLY?

Long before I gave even a second thought to Alzheimer's, I trained Travelers' Aid volunteers at a major airport. It is simply astonishing how people can get themselves into trouble in a strange city—and I have not been immune to doing such foolish things myself. But what surprised me, as I learned the job, was how many people wander through society and some of them are abandoned, left at airports, train or bus stations, hospitals or goodness knows where.

Too many are young and alone with serious problems, but on this subject, I will tell about a typical case, an elderly woman left outside our office in a wheelchair. Oh, she was a handful and her son was easy to find locally, but when he was called to come get her, he said, "I've washed my hands of her. For years I've done everything I could possibly do, and I can't do it anymore." You have to have walked in the shoes of a caregiver to understand that he was probably not a bad son, that he had done all that he could, and one can only do so much for so many years. Maybe she was just a disagreeable old biddy, but if I knew then what I know now, I would have thought she had some type of dementia and too often the caregiver simply burns out and doesn't know what else to do.

The general public has no idea what happens in the privacy of a home when someone has dementia. In bygone years and in many places there still are extended families to help with the caregiving. It is all but impossible for one person to do it all, and too often, that's what happens. A couple, married half a century, still lives in the family home and one gets Alzheimer's. The children and other family members are days away or have died. Who is going to help one elderly spouse take care of the other?

Betty Weiss

Alzheimer's patients wander out in the snow or get lost driving in the desert, often dying. Sometimes they have escaped from a care facility or their own home where they were being properly cared for. In the best of situations there are always some who will fall through the cracks. Who is responsible? The family? The government?

When my husband entered the world of Alzheimer's, I thought that my medical insurance and some government program would pay for things—and they did, but only a little here and there. If you qualify for Medicaid—and each state is different—some might pay for day care, respite and more, even long-term care in a facility or at home. But there are all sorts of qualifications required for most programs, and often one has to spend down assets in order to get assistance. At this point, an elder care attorney can be really important to guide you. Each family is different. Ultimately I bought long-term care insurance for myself; my husband, already diagnosed, would not qualify. If something severe enough happened to me, and our children had to care for both of us, they could soon be bankrupt.

As more people like me are living longer and fewer people are having babies, the demographics make it impossible for the government to take care of everything for everyone. And so Social Security, designed for the population in the 30's, cannot continue to function adequately the same way today.

Most health care programs are set up to help someone who will have treatment then get well, they are not meant to take care of someone who will never get better—year after year after year with something like Alzheimer's. Regulations and restrictions are complex, but generally, with some specific exceptions Medicare, Medicaid, Social Security, private health insurance and HMO's do not cover long-term care. So how do societies care for the elderly who require the greater share of resources but are no longer productive, especially women?

204

While Americans may not treasure the elderly and their wisdom as some societies do, most want the best for their parents. For generations it was the family that took care of their own and many families still embrace that role, but today's smaller families can make that all but impossible. Is it a good thing that filial responsibility is sometimes replaced by the government?

THE WISDOM OF THE ELDERLY

You're going to love this vignette. A young woman I know from India asked if she could talk to me and I said 'sure.' Her Indian fiancée had dumped her and gone back to India at the behest of his mother. She was quite heartbroken, yada, yada and was asking my advice. I told her she was lucky it happened before marriage, that he made his choice to be with his mother in India and not with her. There will be other men. She perked up, smiled and told me, "I knew you'd know how to advise me because you are **old and wise**."

After picking up my teeth, I realized that she meant it as a compliment; Indians revere their elderly and—now hold on—we really are wise. It's not because we are so smart and intelligent, but you can't beat the teacher of life's experience. Most of us have had our hearts broken and broken a few ourselves along the way. *C'est la vie*, been there, done that, survived—life goes on. She's a fast learner. Within days she had a new boyfriend and, as far as I can tell, has never looked back. (Note: I did not relate to my youthful friend the dumb things that I did on my way to becoming so **wise**. Sometimes I remember them, smack myself in the head and wonder how could I have been so **stupid!**)

The whole experience made me think about the way Americans relate to the elderly—that's us, the seniors and oldest old, how other societies behave, and why some are becoming more like us—for good or for bad.

We live with unintended consequences. Because of medical, safety and sanitary advances on many fronts we are living longer. More 'preemies' thrive, fewer women die in childbirth, countless military, accident, burn, drowning and assault victims

206

are saved and repaired, internal bleeding is staunched, limbs are re-attached, the dead are said to have been revived—and more. People survive heart attacks, stroke, cancer; they live with diabetes and other diseases that would have killed them previously. And old age? We have pushed that back substantially.

A male born in 1940 could expect to live 53.9 years, a female, 60.6. Just 50 years later, if born in 1990, a male could expect to live to 72.3 and females 83.6. In 1990 there were 31.0 million Americans over 65, ten years later in 2000, there were 34.9 million and by 2004, there were 36.3 million, a rapidly growing demographic that will impact all of us. Hopefully, most of us will be healthy enough physically and mentally to take care of ourselves for a long time, but realistically, the unintended consequence of all this wonderful life-extending intervention is that more and more of us will develop Alzheimer's or other dementias as we age, need long term care and require a bigger and bigger share of the medical money pie. Life's a gamble, and living longer is a trade-off that few would reject.

My Indian friend said she has never seen an elderly care facility in India like we have here. But I wonder—she was sent here to be educated and graduated from a prestige university with a degree in biology. She has an excellent job, living on her own, although she does speak with her father in India before making major decisions. Will she return to India? Would she easily put aside her social liberties, education and employment to be a family caregiver? Perhaps—she is steeped in filial piety. But could unintended consequences be waiting in the wings?

In my day, a girl's going to college was considered a waste of time since she'd end up being a wife, mother—and ever-the-caretaker for the family. How much education does one need for *that?* Today more females are on campus than males. Will most give up what they worked for to be an unpaid confined caregiver when they can get paid for spending their time at something they enjoy and pay others to care for their loved ones? After all the parental support they gave their daughter through college, will today's Mom and Dad say to give it all up to become their caregiver?

Americans may not revere our elderly, but as a culture we don't discard them. We've never put them on ice floes, sent them into the forest with only a spear, abandoned them on the trail, or expected them to jump on the funeral pyre of their husbands. It is an emotional tearing apart when someone loved is placed in a care facility, an unbearably heart wrenching event and almost always a heavy financial burden. There are exceptions, of course, and to the outsider it may look like it's a carefree choice—that's rarely the case.

NATIONAL CONTACTS
FOR ASSISTANCE

Alzheimer's Association
Phone: 1-800-272-3900*
Phone: 312-335-8700
TTY: 312-335-8882—Fax: 866-669-1246
E-mail: info@alz.org
www.alz.org
Get phone number for the closest Alzheimer's Association office.

National Family Caregivers Association
Phone: 1-800-896-3650*
Phone: 301-942-6430
Fax: 301-492-2302
E-mail: info@thefamilycaregiver.org
www.nfcacares.org

National Association of Professional
Geriatric Care Managers
Phone: 520-881-8008
Fax: 520-325 7925
www.caremanager.org

Family Caregiver Alliance
Phone: 1-800-445-8106*
Phone: 415-434-3388
Fax: 415-434-3508
E-mail: info@caregiver.org
www.caregiver.org

National Alliance for Caregiving
Phone: 301-718-8444
Fax: 301-652-7711
E-mail: info@caregiving.org
www.caregiving.org

National Hospice & Palliative Care Organization
Phone: 1-800-658-8898*
Phone: 703-837-1500
Fax: 703-837-1233
E-mail: nhpco_info@nhpco.org
www.nhpco.org

GOVERNMENT CONTACTS
FOR ASSISTANCE

Administration on Aging
U.S. Department of Health & Human Services
Phone: 202-619-0724
Fax: 202-357-3555
E-mail: aoainfo@aoa.hhs.gov
www.aoa.gov

Centers for Medicare & Medicaid Services
Phone: 1-800-633-4227*
1-877-267-2323*
Phone: 410-786-3000
TTY: 877-486-2048*
www.cms.hhs.gov

Social Security Administration
Phone: 1-800-772-1213*
TTY: 899-325-0778*
www.ssa.gov

Veterans Administration
Phone: 1-800-827-1000*
www.va.gov

*Toll Free Phone Number

YOUR LOCAL CONTACTS
FOR ASSISTANCE

All States and Counties have bureaus for assistance with names like Commission on Aging; Division of Aging & Adult Services; Department of Elder Affairs; Department of Human Services; Division of Senior Citizens.

Phone numbers for such services are found in the front pages of your local phone book under 'Government Listings' for U.S. Government Offices, City, County & State Offices, or use a computer.

Large universities and hospitals often have programs like Memory Clinics; Alzheimer's Research Centers; Aging & Gerontology Centers. Look in your local phone book or on a computer to find such places.

Also look for 'Home Health Services,' 'Nurses' Registries,' 'Mental Health Services.' When caring for someone long distance, look for information in the area where your loved one lives. You never know where any of these contacts may lead.

Information and assistance will not come to you. You will have to find it on your own and it may take many phone calls and conversations before you find the right people. Do not hesitate to ask anywhere for help—doctors, senior centers, senior day care centers, clinics, medical groups, wherever.

SUPPORT GROUPS - FACE-TO-FACE & ON THE COMPUTER

Look for face-to-face support groups. You will learn mountains of valuable information from other participants. Some groups are for the spouse, with or without the other spouse, many are dealing with parents, others are just the general population. Look for support groups at the Alzheimer's Association. Ask at local senior centers. Search the computer for: Alzheimer's Support Groups, Alzheimer's Message Boards, Alzheimer's Chats.

Reach out, help is available.

YOU ARE NOT ALONE!

CPSIA information can be obtained at www.ICGtesting.com
Printed in the USA
LVOW06s0150030114

367869LV00001B/267/P